thefacts

Asthma

also available in thefacts series

the**facts**

Asthma

S. HASAN ARSHAD

School of Medicine
University of Southampton
Southampton
UK

K. SURESH BABU

School of Medicine
University of Southampton
Southampton
UK

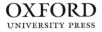
OXFORD
UNIVERSITY PRESS

OXFORD

UNIVERSITY PRESS

Great Clarendon Street, Oxford OX2 6DP

Oxford University Press is a department of the University of Oxford.
It furthers the University's objective of excellence in research, scholarship,
and education by publishing worldwide in

Oxford New York

Auckland Cape Town Dar es Salaam Hong Kong Karachi
Kuala Lumpur Madrid Melbourne Mexico City Nairobi
New Delhi Shanghai Taipei Toronto

With offices in

Argentina Austria Brazil Chile Czech Republic France Greece
Guatemala Hungary Italy Japan Poland Portugal Singapore
South Korea Switzerland Thailand Turkey Ukraine Vietnam

Oxford is a registered trade mark of Oxford University Press
in the UK and in certain other countries

Published in the United States
by Oxford University Press Inc., New York

British Library Cataloguing in Publication Data

Data available

Library of Congress Cataloging in Publication Data
  Arshad, Sayed Hasan.
    Asthma / Sayed Hasan Arshad, K. Suresh Babu.
        p. cm. -- (The facts)
     ISBN 978-0-19-921126-5
1. Asthma--Popular works. I. Babu, K. Suresh, 1968- II. Title.
    RC591.A67 2008
    616.2'38--dc22

                                                            2008024441

ISBN 978-0-19-921126-5

10 9 8 7 6 5 4 3 2 1

Typeset in Plantin
by Cepha Imaging Pvt. Ltd., Bangalore, India
Printed in China
through Asia Pacific Offset Ltd

Foreword

Asthma is a common condition responsible for considerable suffering and healthcare expense. It is one of the few chronic diseases which are becoming more common; currently as many as 1 in 7 children and 1 in 20 adults have active asthma. Treatment, when used correctly, is very effective at suppressing symptoms but it does not cure the condition and most patients will experience recurrent symptoms and will require life-long treatment.

The management of chronic conditions such as asthma has changed radically over the last 20 years. The old 'doctor knows best' approach has been replaced by an approach where management is based on a partnership and dialogue between the patient, his or her carers, and a variety of healthcare professionals. Active invovement of a well-informed patient or carer in treatment decisions is now strongly encouraged by Asthma UK and by many other patient organizations.

How should a patient with asthma or a parent of a child with asthma obtain the necessary background information to participate in decisions on asthma management? Scare stories in newspapers and contradictory and sometimes inaccurate information on the Internet often confuse rather than inform. Against this background a simple, accurate, and accessible book is needed. *Asthma: The Facts* fits the bill admirably. Written by two authors with extensive experience in the management of asthma, the book provides an excellent guide for patients on the cause, classification and treatment of asthma, and useful guidance on the self-management of the condition. I am delighted to provide a foreword for an excellent book, which fills an important gap.

Professor Ian D. Pavord
Consultant Physician and Honorary Professor of Medicine
Glenfield Hospital, Leicester
and Medical Advisor to Asthma UK

Foreword

We are in the midst of a worldwide allergy epidemic. The highest prevalence of all allergic disease occurs in the Western and developed world, with prevalence figures also rising steeply in countries that are adopting a Western-type lifestyle. Asthma and allergy is increasing at an alarming rate (although in the UK it seems to be plateauing at the highest level worldwide). While we have excellent drugs to treat asthma, confusion over how these should be used and relative lack of information about preventative measures means that many patients are not optimally benefitting from recommended asthma management plans.

Asthma: The Facts presents some of the basic principles behind the cause of asthma and its triggers and how this condition in its variable forms can best be managed. What is unique about this book is that it is presented in an easily readable form; 'key points' and 'facts' highlighted throughout the text ensure that the reader can gain easy access to some of the most important principles in terms of asthma's cause, prevention, treatment, and natural history. In addition, the book has useful tables and figures that replace text, instantly providing the reader with essential information.

Asthma is a condition that affects all age groups and can range from the very mildest disease to a life-threatening and complex disorder. As the authors point out, this book helps empower the individual sufferer/patient or the parent of an asthmatic child. It rapidly informs them about the complexity of asthma and what they can do about it. I would like to congratulate the authors for producing such an easily digestible text in a format that I am sure you as a reader will find of great help. I am delighted to be given the privilege of writing this foreword; I do firmly believe that this text will greatly improve the quality of life of many patients with asthma once they have full understanding of the disease and what they can do about it.

Professor Stephen Holgate
Infection, Inflammation and Repair Research Division
School of Medicine
University of Southampton UK

Preface

We feel a sense of achievement in writing this preface because we believe that this book will make a small, but important, contribution towards improved understanding of asthma by patients and parents. This book is written with asthma patients and those involved in their care in mind. The book is part of a series of books aptly named *The Facts;* hence, the name of this book, *Asthma: The Facts.* Let us look at some of the facts relevant to asthma. Asthma affects not millions, but hundreds of millions of children and adults worldwide. Many live in the constant fear of yet another asthma attack. The cost to the economy in many Western countries is enormous and is a major drain on already scarce healthcare resources. The cost of lost school days and productivity is additional to this. The sheer scale of the problem is indeed breathtaking and it is precisely due to this that any effort to improve the lives of asthma patients is likely to have an enormous impact. Moreover, we have excellent management options in asthma, whereby more than 95% of asthma patients should be able to live a completely normal life, with no or minimal symptoms. However, compliance with therapy remains a major problem, and this originates from a lack of understanding of what asthma is and how best to control it. The fact remains that an improved understanding of asthma, its causes, and its management leads to a feeling of self-control and empowerment, and this translates into improved quality of life. Studies have shown that better education and a written management plan can increase compliance and thus overall quality of life for asthma sufferers. Doctors and asthma nurses do their best, but are often limited by their busy schedules. In the UK, we are fortunate to have excellent patient organizations for asthma, such as Asthma UK, which provides education on asthma. This book is not intended to replace these, but to complement information available from these sources. It aims to be a handy reference to provide an overview of the causes of asthma and management options.

The book is presented in a chronological structure; nevertheless, each chapter stands on its own, providing information on one aspect of asthma.

Initially, we have provided a description of the constellation of features that are loosely classed together under the umbrella term of 'asthma', and have tried to explain that asthma has many facets and can indeed present in many different ways. Although everyone knows that asthma is common, some will certainly be interested in finding out exactly how common. The second chapter thus includes some numbers and statistics to explain how common asthma and allergy have become in the early part of the twenty-first century, and speculates on possible reasons. The next chapters explain how asthma affects us and how this effect can be measured objectively. This is followed by chapters describing key aspects of asthma management. We hope that, armed with this knowledge, patients and parents will feel confident to take control of their or their children's asthma. Although many aspects of asthma are common in children and adults, the fact is that children are not small adults. Several features of asthma are specific to children and there are management issues that require special consideration. Therefore, we have devoted Chapter 8 to asthma in childhood. The last chapter covers other allergic diseases that commonly occur in asthmatic patients and which may need to be dealt with in a holistic way.

We firmly believe that doctors should not be prescriptive in the management of chronic diseases such as asthma, but should let the patient have ownership, while empowering them with the knowledge that gives them the confidence to deal with the problem. We hope that this book will do just that, and will find a place at the bedside table of asthma patients and carers. We also hope that they will find this easy to read and will appreciate the fact that it is possible to control asthma, rather than let asthma control their lives.

S. Hasan Arshad

K. Suresh Babu

Contents

1

What is asthma?

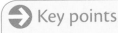 **Key points**

- Asthma is a long-term disease that affects the breathing tubes that carry air in and out of the lungs

- Childhood allergic asthma is more common in boys than in girls

- Around one in ten cases of asthma in adults is due to occupational exposure to allergens

- Estimates vary, but aspirin sensitivity may occur in 5–10% of asthmatics

Asthma is a common disease that affects approximately 300 million children and adults worldwide. It is so common that it is now regarded as a serious public health problem. Asthma may be mild, in which case it does not cause a great deal of concern. However, in other situations, it may be a serious and even life-threatening condition. Caring for people with asthma is time-consuming and expensive. The global burden of asthma is increasing, particularly in children, leading to increasing healthcare costs, reductions in quality of life, and increased take-up of hospital beds for management of asthma attacks. How asthma is managed depends upon the individual's understanding of asthma, which determines the level of control, the need for emergency visits, and the number of school/work days lost. A better understanding of asthma by patients and parents is paramount in improving the quality of life and in reducing hospital admissions by recognizing the early warning signs of worsening asthma.

What is asthma?

Asthma is a chronic disease that affects the breathing tubes that carry air in and out of the lungs. The airways are inflamed (swollen) in asthma, and this makes them very twitchy and sensitive. A sensitive airway reacts to various different irritants causing narrowing, leading to reduced airflow through the lungs. The narrowing of the airways is due to a combination of increased secretions within the airways as a consequence of inflammation and to the constriction of the muscles around the airways (Figure 1.1). This manifests as:

- wheezing (a whistling noise while breathing);
- chest tightness;
- cough;
- breathing difficulties.

These symptoms are more common during the night and early morning. Wheezing is the sound that is heard when air tries to escape from the narrowed breathing tubes. Symptoms are variable from individual to individual, but do get worse during an asthma attack, which is usually caused by an infection, exposure to allergens, or other factors leading to an inability to expel air from the lungs.

The factors or triggers for asthma vary from individual to individual. A trigger is anything that sets off an asthma attack. Common triggers for asthma are shown in Table 1.1.

Types of asthma

Previously, it was thought that asthma has two main subtypes, i.e. allergic (also called extrinsic) asthma and non-allergic (also called intrinsic) asthma.

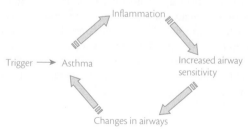

Figure 1.1 The asthma cycle.

Table 1.1 Asthma triggers

Trigger	Examples
Allergen	House dust mite, animals (cat and dog), cockroaches, pollen, trees, mould
Infection	Virus infections such as coughs and colds
Pollutants	Cigarette smoke (active or passive), sulphur dioxide
Occupational agents	Flour, certain chemicals
Foods	Seafood, nuts, food additives such as sulphites
Drugs	Heart drugs (atenolol, propranolol, bisoprolol), pain killers (ibuprofen, voltarol)
Psychological factors	Stress, anxiety, intense emotions
Cold air	
Exercise	
Hyperventilation	
Others	Chemical agents, perfumes, etc.

However, there are various types of asthma with considerable overlap between these two categories. In fact, asthma is best regarded not as one disease, but as a multifaceted condition, where one or more aspects, often in varying combinations, are evident in any one individual. This will become apparent as we read more about asthma types in the following sections.

Allergic asthma

Individuals whose asthma symptoms are brought about by exposure to one or more allergens are said to have allergic asthma. Overall, this is the commonest form and is particularly common in children (60–70% of asthma in children is allergic asthma). This is also called atopic asthma. Atopy is an inherited tendency in some individuals to produce a particular type of antibody called immunoglobulin E or IgE for short. These antibodies are produced when someone is exposed to a new allergen for the first time or the first few times in life (called the initial exposure). Once these antibodies have been produced, they have the ability to react on subsequent exposures to the same allergen.

The reaction that ensues in the body following these subsequent exposures may produce the symptoms of asthma. It is possible to identify what these individuals with allergic asthma might react to by doing an allergy skin test. When a suspected allergen is injected under their skin, these individuals react with localized itching, swelling, and redness. Those with a hereditary tendency towards this type of allergy are likely to have allergic asthma, but in addition may develop a number of other related allergic conditions such as hay fever, runny nose (rhinitis), eczema, hives, and skin rashes.

 Fact!

Childhood allergic asthma is more common in boys than in girls.

Avoidance of specific allergens (for example, those identified by an allergy skin test) and other precipitating factors is helpful in the management of asthma.

Non-allergic asthma

In a subgroup of asthmatics, allergens do not play a significant role in causing asthma symptoms or asthma attacks. These are patients who often develop asthma in adulthood, and an allergy skin test or blood test cannot identify a specific allergen. The allergy antibody (IgE) levels are low in these groups. What causes asthma in these individuals remains a mystery and it is difficult to identify a triggering agent. Nonetheless, inhalation of chemicals and cigarette smoke, exposure to cold air, laughter, food additives, and a myriad of other factors are implicated and may act as an irritant in the bronchial tubes.

In common with patients with allergic asthma, these people have twitchy airways and manifest symptoms such as wheezing, chest tightness, and cough. This group does not need to worry about avoidance of allergens such as dust mites or furry animals. However, avoidance of irritant triggers such as cigarette smoke, perfumes, and cold air should be possible and does help.

Exercise-induced asthma

Physical exertion is an important cause of symptoms in many patients with asthma. For some people, exercise is the only cause of their asthma symptoms. These subjects do not usually have any symptoms until they exercise, when symptoms of breathing difficulty, a sense of tightness in the chest, and wheezing (a whistling sound) develop. Symptoms rarely occur during exercise; they more typically develop 5–10 minutes after completing the exercise. Symptoms vary in severity and in most cases resolve within 30–45 minutes. Children with exercise-induced asthma are not able to keep up with their peers in games and thus avoid participation in physical activities. Exercise-induced asthma is more common in younger people, and it is believed that the airways of these patients are sensitive to changes in the temperature and humidity of the air.

In cold, dry weather, the effect of exercise is exaggerated. When at rest, we breathe through the nose, which warms and humidifies the air making it more like the air in the lungs, but while exercising, we breathe through our mouth, making the air delivered to the lungs colder and dryer. This difference between the warm air in the lungs and the cold, dry inhaled air can trigger asthmatic symptoms. Once triggered, the muscles around the bronchial tubes constrict and the lining of the breathing tubes swells, leading to narrowing and asthma symptoms.

Some forms of exercise such as running are more likely to precipitate asthma symptoms. Sports and games that require more continuous activity and those that are played in cold weather are more likely to precipitate exercise-induced asthma. These include:

- long-distance running;

- basketball;

- ice and field hockey;

- football;

- cross-country skiing.

Activities that are less likely to trigger asthma symptoms include:

- walking;

- swimming;

- track and field events;

- golf;

- volleyball;

- wrestling;

- gymnastics;

- hiking.

The severity of symptoms depends upon the individual's sensitivity, how cold or dry the ambient air is (the colder and drier the air, the more severe the symptoms), if the exercise is continuous or intermittent (the symptoms are more severe with continuous exercise), and how strenuous the exercise is (the more strenuous it is, the greater the need to breathe more heavily and therefore the more severe the symptoms). Taking prophylactic medications can prevent the onset of symptoms, and allow children to participate in games and healthy physical activities.

Cough-variant asthma

In some individuals with asthma, chronic (long-term) cough is the principal, if not the only, symptom of asthma. This is more common in children and the symptoms are more pronounced at night. The cough is usually dry or non-productive. These patients usually do not have the typical symptoms of wheezing, chest tightness, or shortness of breath. However, they may have hypersensitivity of the airways as in patients with typical asthma and they may react to triggers such as exercise, exposure to allergens, and irritants. Cough-variant asthma should not be considered as a different entity because there is inflammation of the airways in this group similar to that of typical asthma. However, when these patients present with cough as the only symptom, it is important to consider other causes of chronic cough.

The diagnosis of cough-variant asthma is difficult. These patients do not have typical asthma symptoms such as wheezing or difficulty breathing, and often have normal lung function. Apart from excluding other causes of chronic cough, it is important to make a positive diagnosis of asthma. This can be done with certain tests. These patients may manifest hypersensitivity of the airways, which can be demonstrated using specialized breathing tests. A treatment response may also be of help. For example, administration of bronchodilators or steroid-containing inhalers may improve the symptoms, indicating the presence of an underlying tendency towards asthma. Once the diagnosis is made, it is important to treat this group of patients, because 30% of patients with cough-variant asthma eventually develop classical asthma.

Nocturnal asthma

Nocturnal asthma is a term used to describe the asthma of patients whose symptoms get worse at night. It is still being debated whether nocturnal asthma is a separate type of asthma or is only a symptom of severe asthma. The majority of these patients—almost 75%—experience increased symptoms at night, and frequent night-time wakening due to asthma implies poor asthma control. The breathing problems associated with nocturnal asthma often cause patients to awaken during the night.

Disruption of the amount or quality of sleep can result in daytime sleepiness, and may affect the ability to learn and perform tasks. Therefore, treatment for nocturnal asthma can improve the quality of life for these patients. The signs and symptoms of nocturnal asthma are similar to classical asthma, but are often under-reported because they occur at night. This indicates that nocturnal asthma may merely reflect poor control of asthma, and this is perhaps the case in the majority of people with prominent asthma symptoms at night. However, some patients do not have severe asthma and have hardly any symptoms during the daytime, but are bothered by symptoms, often chronic cough, at night. These patients may be suffering from a variant form of asthma.

 Fact!

The majority of nocturnal asthma symptoms occur between midnight and 8 a.m., peaking at 4 a.m.

It is at this time of night that the lung functions are at their lowest levels. This is mainly due to normal variations in the body functions that facilitate changes according to the time of day (or night), something called circadian rhythm. It is partly explained by the level of certain hormones such as adrenalin and cortisol, which are at their lowest levels during the early morning hours. These hormones are protective against asthma, as their natural effect is to widen the airways and suppress inflammation.

Other factors may also explain the occurrence of nocturnal symptoms in asthma. Some argue that exposure to the house dust mite may be an explanation in those who are sensitized to this allergen. House dust mite allergen is found in abundance in mattresses and pillows, and even minor disturbances of this reserve as we sleep increases the level of allergen in the air that we breath during the night.

Other factors such as reduced levels of asthma medication in the body system at night and a decrease in room temperature may also play a part. Another factor in some people may be acid reflux (heartburn), which can make asthma worse at night. In the lying position, stomach acids may trickle back into the throat and then into our breathing tubes or airways. The lining of the airways is very sensitive, and even the tiniest amount of acid irritates and burns the lining, initiating a cough response; this may become persistent if this acid trickling occurs every night or on a regular basis. It can then lead to chronic inflammation seen in the more typical forms of asthma (as opposed to nocturnal cough only). Successful treatment of the heartburn can sometimes improve asthma symptoms. Nocturnal asthma appears more often in patients who are obese. The reason for this is not entirely clear, but may be related to increase acid reflux or hormonal effects.

Occupational asthma

Occupational asthma is defined as asthma caused by exposure to an agent encountered in the work environment. Over 300 substances have been associated with occupational asthma. These include:

- small molecules such as isocyanates;

- irritants;

- platinum salts;

- animal biological products;

- plant products.

These are all capable of provoking the immune system to produce allergic antibody (IgE). Occupational asthma generally affects adults of working age as they become exposed to sensitizing chemicals at their work place.

 Fact!

Around one in ten cases of asthma in adults is due to occupational exposure to allergens.

Individuals working in certain types of work or industry are at higher risk. These include:

- farming and agricultural work;

- painting (including spray painting);

- cleaning work;

- plastic manufacturing.

Soldering is a procedure that is used commonly in many industries, particularly in the electronic industry. Certain resins used as flux in soldering may give rise to vapours of a substance called colophony, which is an important cause of occupational asthma. Substances of biological origin, such as flour, wood dust, and animal dander, are also important causes of both occupational asthma and occupational rhinitis.

Table 1.2 Suspected causes of occupational asthma

Substance	Industry/occupation at risk
Isocyanates	Polyurethane: insulators, laminators; plastics: roofers, painters, chemists, rubber workers
Anhydrides	Chemical workers, paint and plastic workers, those working with epoxy resins
Metals	Chrome platers, welders, platinum refiners, nickel platers, tool grinders, diamond polishers
Drugs	Pharmaceuticals, laboratory workers, farm workers, fumigators, pesticide formulators
Formaldehyde	Embalmers, laboratory workers, insulators, textile workers
Glutaraldehyde	Hospital staff
Ethylenediamine	Photographic processors, rubber workers
Persulfate salts	Beauticians, chemical workers
Ammonium thioglycolate	Beauticians
Hexamethylenamine	Pesticide industry
Polyvinyl chloride	Meat wrappers
Pyrethrin	Fumigators
Animals	Farmers, veterinarians, meat processing, poultry breeders, bird fanciers, laboratory workers, oyster farmers, prawn and crab processors, silk sericulturers
Plants	Farmers, grain handlers, bakers, brewers, millers, textile workers, cigarette manufacturers, spice processors, coffee and castor bean workers
Vegetable gums	Printing, food processing
Wood dusts	Woodworkers
Dyes	Fabric and fur dyeing, cosmetics, dye manufacturers
Fluxes (Colophony)	Solderers, electronic workers
Enzymes	Pharmaceutical workers, detergent manufacturers, food processors, plastic and rubber workers

People working in these environments do not become asthmatic as soon as they start work and are exposed to these chemical or biological substances. Indeed, it is not uncommon for asthma to appear months or even years after the onset of exposure to the sensitizing substance. Why some people develop occupational asthma whilst others, working in the same environment, do not is not entirely clear. However, it may depend on their genetic risk in combination with other environmental exposures. For example, individuals with an inherited allergic tendency (atopy) are at higher risk. Similarly, those who smoke run a higher risk of becoming sensitized to these occupational substances and developing asthma.

Workers may be unaware of the possible relationship between their symptoms and their work. Even if they do suspect a link, they may still be reluctant to present their concerns to their doctor, fearing adverse consequences for their employment. The indicators of occupational asthma include development or worsening of asthma-type symptoms at work or after work, with disturbance of sleep and an improvement in symptoms when away from work (for example, over the weekend or while on holiday). The symptoms are the same as those of more typical forms of asthma, including wheezing, chest tightness, cough, chest pain, shortness of breath, and fatigue. These symptoms may or may not be associated with rhinitis (hay fever)-type symptoms such as sneezing, a stuffy runny nose, and itchy eyes indicating the presence of occupational rhinitis, or itchy red skin (indicating occupational eczema).

> Once a diagnosis of occupational asthma has been established, complete avoidance of the sensitizer is paramount in the management of this condition.

If diagnosis and avoidance of the sensitizer is carried out early enough, it is likely that asthma symptoms will improve quickly and may even disappear. However, if exposure to the substance had continued for some time, the disease may persist for several years, even after removal from exposure of the causative agent. Continued exposure may lead to increasingly severe and potentially fatal asthma exacerbations. Some of the occupations that can lead to occupational asthma are listed in Table 1.2.

Aspirin-sensitive asthma

Most people with asthma do not have any problems with aspirin. However, some subjects with asthma develop symptoms if they consume aspirin or other related painkillers (non-steroidal anti-inflammatory drugs).

> Estimates vary, but aspirin sensitivity may occur in 5–10% of asthmatics.

Often, patients with asthma are advised by their physicians to avoid aspirin in case they have aspirin sensitivity. This is because there is no simple test to confirm or refute this possibility. If asthma symptoms clearly get worse or someone has an exacerbation after taking aspirin, then aspirin and non-steroidal anti-inflammatory drugs should be avoided. If there is any doubt, an inhalation test (called an aspirin-lysine bronchial challenge) can be organized by an asthma specialist.

 ## Case study

Asthma and sensitivity to aspirin

A 24-year-old man developed nettle rash after taking aspirin for a headache. The rash and swelling subsided over the next few hours, but a couple of weeks later he had another similar episode after taking aspirin. He avoided aspirin, but over the next few weeks, he gradually developed an intermittent rash and the respiratory symptoms of cough, wheezing, shortness of breath, and chest tightness. He could not identify any specific triggers for these symptoms. He made an appointment with his GP who, after assessment, told him that he had developed asthma and needed treatment with inhalers. With regular use of a preventative inhaler, he improved, but some wheezing and rash persisted. He was referred to an asthma specialist who, after assessment, made a diagnosis of aspirin sensitivity causing asthma and recurrent urticaria (rash) was made. He was put on a diet that excluded food containing small quantities of salicylate for four weeks. His symptoms improved significantly, and his requirement for the rescue inhaler was reduced. He was then asked to reintroduce salicylate, and, within a week, his rash and asthma symptoms returned, confirming the diagnosis.

Refractory asthma

In characterizing the severity of asthma, various factors need to be considered including:

- the level of symptoms and medication use;

- pulmonary function;

- the degree of sensitivity of the airways;

- the type and severity of airway inflammation;

- the need for hospitalization;

◆   the frequency and severity of exacerbations;

◆   the response to treatment;

◆   the impact on health and well-being.

> Refractory asthma is defined as asthma with persistent symptoms and/or frequent or serious exacerbations accompanied by serious airway obstruction that requires high doses of steroids to control.

Other equivalent designations are severe or difficult-to-control asthma. This is only a small proportion (5–10%) of the total number of asthmatics, but they account for the majority of hospital admissions and hospital visits for asthma worsening. These patients do have certain features peculiar to this form of asthma, such as a specific type of inflammation in the airways. Nonetheless, it is not clear whether this is a distinct form of asthma or simply typical asthma that is very severe. The important aspect of labelling someone with refractory asthma is that these individuals should be managed by a specialist. It is also imperative that they adhere to their prescribed medications, avoid smoking, and are aware of the early symptoms of asthma worsening for early intervention.

Steroid-resistant asthma

A prominent feature of asthma is the presence of inflammation in the airways. This inflammation almost always responds to treatment with steroids, usually given in inhaled form, but occasionally as tablets or injections, e.g. during an attack or for those with severe asthma. A minority of those with severe asthma do not respond adequately even to oral steroids. These patients are regarded as having steroid-resistant asthma. Whether this lack of response to steroids is simply a manifestation of the severity of asthma or is indeed a separate entity is not clear.

Does smoking cause asthma?

The answer to the question of whether asthma can be caused by smoking is not straightforward. Smoking usually causes chronic bronchitis and emphysema, which are different diseases. However, some people with chronic bronchitis and emphysema do behave like asthmatics. Moreover, some people with asthma, when they smoke, develop a mixed type of disease with features of both asthma and bronchitis/emphysema. There is also evidence that smoking may increase the risk of asthma developing in the first place.

Research has revealed that people whose partners smoke are nearly five times more likely to develop asthma than those who are not exposed to passive smoking.

It is also believed that children of mothers who smoked during pregnancy are more likely to have respiratory problems and are much more likely to develop asthma. Children are especially at risk because their lungs are smaller and still developing. Exposure to second-hand smoke can lead to decreased lung function and symptoms of airway inflammation. These people are also more likely to develop lung and sinus infections. These infections can make asthma symptoms worse and more difficult to control.

There is no doubt that exposure to cigarette smoke makes asthma symptoms worse, whether it is active (by the asthmatic subject) or passive (by those around them). Because the airways of asthmatics are more sensitive than non-asthmatic subjects, smoking irritates the airways of asthmatic subjects even more, making them inflamed, swollen, narrow, and full of mucus. This leads to worsening symptoms of asthma such as cough, wheezing, and shortness of breath. These symptoms are similar to those during an asthma flare-up. In other words, smoking can lead to frequent asthma flare-ups, which may be more severe and more difficult to control, even with medication.

Studies have shown that asthma control is significantly worse in asthmatics who smoke compared with those who have never smoked, with all symptoms related to asthma control uniformly worse in smokers, even in those with relatively good lung function. Furthermore, smoking can reduce the effect of any controlling medications being taken for asthma and can increase the use of rescue medications. Inhaled steroids are the mainstay of treatment in asthma acting as preventers of symptoms. Smoking confers a degree of steroid resistance in asthma, thereby making the drugs less efficacious. In addition, the long-term effect of smoking in asthmatics is to cause permanent damage to their lungs and airways.

Quitting smoking and avoiding second-hand smoke therefore:

- improves asthma control;

- improves asthma flare-ups;

- decreases the number of emergency visits to hospital;

- improves the response to medications, both preventative and rescue;

- reduces the likelihood of developing asthma in adulthood;

- decreases the likelihood of asthma persisting in adulthood.

There is evidence to suggest that by the sixth week after ceasing smoking, there is considerable improvement in lung function and a reduction in the inflammation of the airways compared with individuals who continue to smoke, highlighting the importance of smoking cessation in asthma patients.

Classification of asthma severity

Asthma is classified into various categories based primarily on the level and frequency of symptoms, i.e. whether symptoms are mild, moderate, or severe, and if these symptoms are intermittent or persistent.

> The four categories of asthma are mild intermittent, mild persistent, moderate persistent, and severe persistent.

The degree of impairment of lung function is also taken into account (Table 1.3).

The classification of asthma is useful for decision-making in asthma management. This classification of asthma according to severity reflects not only the severity of the underlying disease, but also the responsiveness to treatment and is subject to change. For example, on initial presentation, an individual could be classified as having severe persistent asthma, but could respond well to treatment and then be reclassified as having moderate persistent asthma.

Table 1.3 Classification of asthma

Category	Symptoms
Intermittent	Symptoms less than once a week
	Occasional, mild, and short-lasting exacerbations
	Night-time symptoms less than twice a month
	Good lung function, as indicated by:
	◆ FEV_1 or PEF more than 80% of normal or expected
	◆ variation in FEV_1 or PEF of less than 20%
Mild persistent	Symptoms more than once a week, but less than once a day
	Exacerbations may affect sleep and activities
	Night-time symptoms more than twice a month
	Average lung function, as indicated by:
	◆ FEV_1 or PEF more than 80% of normal or expected
	◆ variation in FEV_1 or PEF of 20–30%
Moderate persistent	Daily symptoms
	Exacerbations may affect sleep and activities
	Night-time symptoms more than once a week

(continued)

Table 1.3 Classification of asthma (*continued*)

Category	Symptoms
	◆ FEV$_1$ or PEF 60–80% of normal or expected
	◆ variation in FEV$_1$ or PEF of more than 30%
Severe persistent	Daily symptoms
	Frequent exacerbations
	Frequent night-time symptoms
	Limitations of physical activity
	Poor lung function, as indicated by:
	◆ FEV$_1$ or PEF of less than 60% of normal or expected
	◆ variation in FEV$_1$ or PEF of more than 30%

PEF, peak expiratory flow; FEV$_1$, forced expiratory volume in one second

Lung function tests or pulmonary function tests evaluate how well the lungs work. The simplest breathing test is called peak expiratory flow (PEF), which is a measure of how rapidly the patient can blow out air. This is directly related to the size of the bronchial tubes, which tend to narrow in asthma. A variation in the size of bronchial tubes causing changes in peak flow is one of the main features of asthma and helps in the diagnosis. Spirometry is also a basic lung function test. It measures how much and how quickly a person can move air out of the lungs. For this test, after a deep breath, the person is asked to breathe forcefully into a mouthpiece attached to a recording device (spirometer), and various volumes of air are recorded and can be printed. The most useful is FEV$_1$ (forced expiratory volume in one second), i.e. the amount of air that comes out in the first second of a forceful breathing effort. Other parameters are also sometimes measured to assess detailed lung function, severity of airway narrowing, and the twitchiness of the airways. These will be dealt with in subsequent chapters.

2

Is asthma increasing?

 Key points

- Asthma is the most common chronic disease in children

- There has been an increase of severalfold in the prevalence of asthma and allergy over the last few decades

- There are several genes that predispose to asthma and allergy

- Both genes and environment contribute to the development of asthma

How common is asthma?

In recent decades, asthma has become a very common condition. Previous to this, in a class of 25 children, we would have expected to see at most one child with asthma. It is now not uncommon to find several children in any one class who are asthmatic or who use an asthma inhaler before their regular physical activity period. It has been estimated that, in developed countries, between 5 and 10% of the total population now suffer from asthma. Asthma occurs more frequently in children, with approximately one in seven children suffering from the condition. These estimates are fairly reliable because they originate from studies using standardized and validated criteria for diagnosis. Occupational asthma constitutes 9–15% of all adult-onset asthma and is the most commonly reported occupational disease in the developed world. In children, asthma is more common in boys than in girls, but this reverses in adults where asthma is more common in women than men (about 60% of adults with asthma are women).

Variations in the prevalence of asthma

Although asthma occurs in all populations across the world, it does not occur with the same frequency in every country. Indeed, there is a huge variation in the prevalence of asthma and wheezing (Figure 2.1). When studies were carried out using the same methodology and diagnostic criteria, it was found that asthma was more common in the developed world. The highest prevalence was observed in English-speaking countries such as the UK, Australia, and New Zealand. Countries with a low prevalence included eastern European countries, Albania, Greece, China, Taiwan, Uzbekistan, India, Indonesia, and Ethiopia.

Interestingly, surveys in developing countries show that asthma is more prevalent in cities than in rural areas. In Kenya, for example, asthma is virtually unknown in villages, yet it is increasingly being seen in the cities. However, in developed countries, there is no difference between rural and urban asthma prevalence. In addition, first-generation immigrant populations moving from developing to developed countries keep their low risk of asthma, whilst the second generation, born and brought up in the West, seem quickly to acquire a higher risk for asthma. Why urbanization and Westernization should make a difference to asthma risk will be discussed later in this chapter.

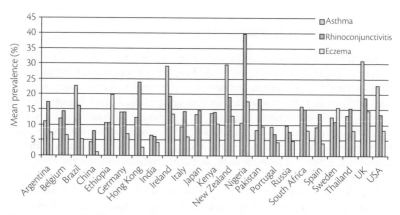

Figure 2.1 Worldwide prevalence of asthma, rhinoconjunctivitits, and eczema. Created with data from 'Worldwide time trends in the prevalence of symptoms of asthma, allergic rhinoconjunctivitis, and eczema in childhood: ISAAC Phases One and Three repeat multicountry cross-sectional surveys', Asher, M.I., Montefort, S., Björkstén, B., et al. (2006) The Lancet 368, pp. 733–743.

Increasing prevalence of asthma

From the above discussion, we can safely conclude that the prevalence of asthma is high, at least in the developed world. If we go back to the 1940s and 1950s, we know that the prevalence of asthma was not this high. Do the recent estimates truly indicate a rise in the prevalence of asthma in recent decades or is this merely a function of increased awareness and better diagnostic methods? For example, some argue that renaming terms such as 'bronchitis' as asthma may have contributed to the recent high-prevalence estimates. There is probably some truth in this. However, there is also good evidence to support the view that there has been an actual rise in the prevalence of asthma. The irrefutable evidence comes from repeated studies carried out several years or decades apart, in the same population, and using the same methodology and diagnostic criteria.

Asthma statistics

In the USA:

◆ asthma affects almost 17 million people;

◆ there has been a 75% increase in the last 20 years;

◆ 1 in 13 children and 1 in 20 adults may have asthma;

◆ since 1980, asthma in children under 5 years has risen by 160% and in school-aged children by 75%.

In the UK:

◆ 1 in 7 children has asthma (compared with approximately 1 in 50 in the late 1970s);

◆ overall, 5.2 million British people suffer from asthma;

◆ the number of adults with asthma has increased by 400,000 from 2001 to 2006;

◆ the number of children in whom asthma was diagnosed at some point in their life increased from 5.5 to 12% between 1964 and 1989 (and has more than doubled to 27% in 2003).

However, recent data in some countries indicate that this rise in the prevalence of asthma may now have stabilized. The indications were first noticed in the late 1990s when it was shown that the rate of hospitalization for asthma, which went up with the rise in prevalence during the 1980s, seemed to have plateaued followed by a slight decline. Initially, this improvement was thought to be due to better diagnostics, improved treatments (especially the increased use of inhaled steroids), and better education about asthma in the 1990s. There is certainly a significant element of this. However, some recent data from Canada confirm that not only has the rate of hospitalization and attendance at Accident and Emergency departments decreased, but the diagnosis of asthma in the population has also stabilized.

Asthma and allergy

The rise in the prevalence of asthma has been mirrored, to some extent, by other allergic diseases such as allergic rhinitis (hay fever), allergic or atopic eczema, and food allergies. This is not unexpected, because asthma and allergy often coexist. The majority of asthma is allergic and therefore those with allergic asthma may also have other allergic diseases. So, what is the connection between asthma and allergy?

What is allergy?

Allergy is a term that is commonly used loosely to indicate an aversion to something. We often hear people saying that they are allergic to a place or a person or even 'Monday mornings'. However, in scientific terms, allergy is an over-reaction of the immune system, causing harmful effects, to something that is normally harmless, such as pollen or peanuts. When this allergic reaction occurs in the airways, an inflammatory response follows. If the allergen exposure occurs on most days or every day, for example an allergy to dust mites, it produces chronic inflammation of the airways—the hallmark of asthma. Similar process occurring in the nose and eyes may cause hay fever during summer.

 Fact!

Allergy is a reaction that may occur anywhere in the body, whilst asthma is a condition that is produced when this reaction occurs in the airways.

It can be assumed that allergy or allergic diseases are even more common than asthma, because allergy would include not only allergic asthma, but also other types of allergic reaction and disease. Atopy (being allergic as a result of hereditary factors) is the single strongest risk factor for the development of asthma (and, of course, allergy), increasing the risk by 10–20-fold compared with those who are non-allergic.

Allergens

Allergens are biological substances, i.e. originating from plants or animals, such as pollen, dust mites, or foods. Common allergens include aeroallergens (those we inhale), food allergens (those we eat), and those injected through

the skin (drugs, insect venom, etc.) (see Table 2.1). A number of factors
determine which allergen causes what type of symptoms. Prominent among
these factors are the characteristics of the allergen and how it enters the body.
For example, food allergens usually cause oral symptoms, vomiting, and skin
rashes, and occasionally more severe reactions involving many parts of the
body, a reaction known as anaphylaxis. Insect allergens entering through the
skin as the result of a sting (like an injection) may cause a localized reaction or,
if severe, may cause anaphylaxis. On the other hand, allergens that are inhaled,
such as house dust mites, cause respiratory allergy (asthma or hay fever).

Table 2.1 Common allergens

Type	Allergen
Outdoor aeroallergens	Pollens ◆ grasses ◆ trees ◆ weeds ◆ flowers Animals ◆ horse ◆ rabbit
Indoor aeroallergens	House dust mite Cockroaches Moulds ◆ Aspergillus ◆ Candida ◆ Alternaria ◆ Cladosporium
Food allergens	Cows' milk Egg Peanut and tree nuts Fish and shellfish
Drugs	Antibiotics Anaesthetic agents Aspirin and other analgesics
Other	Latex, insects, dyes, etc.

How common is allergy?

The prevalence of allergy at any one time in the UK is estimated to be around 20% and, in any one year, 12 million people are likely to seek treatment for allergic problems. It is well known that children suffer from allergies more than adults and that allergies often peak during adolescence. In the UK, a survey of 13–14-year-old children showed that up to 32% reported symptoms of asthma, 9% had eczema, and 40% could have allergic rhinitis (hay fever). Allergic disease affects both sexes, and all ethnic and social groups.

 Fact!

An estimated 50 million Americans suffer from one or more allergic conditions.

All allergy-related conditions have shown a rise in recent years including:

* asthma;

* allergic rhinitis and atopic eczema;

* food allergies;

* systemic allergic reactions to:
  * latex;
  * insect stings;
  * drugs.

Again, this increase has been shown primarily in Western, developed countries, but developing countries with increasing urbanization are not far behind. Allergy prevalence overall has been increasing since the early 1960s across all age, sex, and racial groups. Just like asthma, studies have been repeated in the same areas, using the same validated methods, and have shown that this increase in, for example, allergic rhinitis or nut allergy is real and not merely due to changes in definition or awareness.

Allergy and heredity

Allergies have a strong hereditary component. If only one parent has allergies of one kind or another, the chances are one in three that their child will be allergic. If both parents have allergies, it is much more likely (seven out of ten children) that their children will have allergies. The same allergy is transferred from parents to children more than a different allergic disease. For example, if parents have asthma, the child is more likely to have asthma and less likely to have eczema or hay fever, although their chance of developing one of these diseases is still higher than that of a child whose parents do not have any allergic disease.

Fact!

The risk of a child developing asthma is higher if the mother has asthma than if the father suffers from the disease. Why this should be so is not clear.

Genes and asthma

Asthma tends to run in families. We often see many people with asthma in one family, perhaps spread over generations, indicating the genetic effect. However, this hereditary effect is not simple. In other words, even if both parents have asthma, the child will not necessarily have asthma, despite having an increased risk. Sometimes a generation is missed, i.e. a child and a grandparent may have asthma whilst there is no asthma in either parent. Studies of twins are interesting and in the early days of genetic research, they provided the strongest proof that genetic factors contribute importantly to asthma. Identical twins, who have almost the same genes, tend to behave similarly with regard to asthma (as with many other characteristics controlled by genes), i.e. the likelihood that both will have asthma, or that neither will, is very high. When twins are non-identical (these twins only share genes to the same degree as any other siblings would), the likelihood is high, but not very high.

Asthma genes

We now know that asthma is caused by not one gene, but probably a large number of genes. Each gene has only a small effect, but in the right combination they increase the risk sufficiently to cause the disease. However, the specific combination of genes that causes asthma is being investigated. There is probably not one, but several (or several hundred!) different combinations that will eventually be identified as the genetic make-up of a child who will develop asthma. This is called polygenic heritability, i.e. many distinct genes are involved. To date, several genes have been identified as being associated with asthma and they are widely spread over different areas of the human genome. This may be a reflection of the complicated nature of asthma, as in real life we see asthma presenting itself in many different ways (see Chapter 1). Despite this complication, the study of genes is very important, because it can tell us exactly who is likely to suffer from asthma, who will respond to the different types of treatment, and may also help scientists to devise new and more effective treatments.

Genes and the environment

Although the identification of asthma genes is still in its early stages, the genetic findings are changing the prevailing view of asthma. For example, one study showed that genetic factors may determine how the lining of the airways develop with very minute defects that allow relatively easy entry of allergens. Of course, the child may need to have some genes for allergy as well to be able to respond to the allergens in a specific way. Hence, it may be that both asthma and allergy genes are required. A further layer of complication is added with the role of environment factors. Thus, a typical scenario can be described in which:

- the person may have asthma genes and hence the airways have developed in a certain way;

- they may also have allergy genes and thus may become allergic to common allergens such as the house dust mite; and

- the individual will also need to be exposed to the relevant allergens— hence, the effect of the environment in the development of asthma.

 Fact!

Exposure to indoor and some outdoor allergens is an important risk factor for the development of asthma and allergic disease.

Asthma and the environment

In addition to the genetic effect, environmental exposure is also of primary importance for the occurrence and development of allergic diseases, including asthma, as mentioned above. This importance is evidenced by several observations. The fact that asthma has increased severalfold in the last few decades is testimony to this. Although genes can change with evolution, this occurs, as a rule, over several hundred or thousand years. Our genes do not change significantly over 30–40 years. Thus, the increase in asthma and allergic disease must be due to environmental changes. Moreover, variations in the prevalence of asthma around the globe also underscore the importance of the environment. Differences in genetics among populations are usually minor, whereas differences in environmental exposure can be huge.

Environmental factors

Common environmental factors include:

- diet;

- infection;

- allergens;

- pollution.

Environmental exposure is shared by children living in the same family and thus contributes to sibling similarity in the occurrence of asthma (in addition to common genes). Such shared environmental exposure includes the type of diet, parental smoking, air pollution, domestic animals, and other allergens such as dust mites, cockroaches, and moulds. In other words, rather than inheriting asthma itself, we inherit a tendency to develop asthma, and this inherited tendency will only come to fruition if we are also exposed to the environmental stimuli that trigger asthma.

Occupational exposure

Further evidence for the development of asthma as a result of environmental factors comes from occupational exposure. Occupational exposure to various chemicals and other substances occurs on a regular, repeated, and long-term basis. A number of chemicals have sensitizing properties and, after regular inhalation, some people develop allergies to these chemicals leading to the development of asthma. Chemicals such as diisocyanates (used, for example, in spray painting) are strong allergens that can cause asthma symptoms in sensitized individuals at very low concentrations and have even been responsible for a few deaths due to asthma. Not everyone working in these environments and exposed to these chemicals develops occupational asthma. Why only some individuals develop asthma on exposure to the offending agent is not clear, but is possibly due to their genetic make-up.

Pollution and asthma

Few issues raise political and emotional feelings as much as the effect of air pollution on health. However, it has proved difficult to establish that asthma is caused by pollution. Some epidemiological observations do suggest that this might be so. For example, urbanization has been associated with a higher prevalence of asthma. With urbanization comes air pollution from industry and road traffic. There is also experimental observation that inhalation of pollutants may increase the risk of allergen sensitization and the development of

Table 2.2 Pollution levels on the Isle of Wight

National air quality objectives		Estimate for Isle of Wight (mg/m^3)
Pollutant	**Concentration (mg/m^3)**	
Benzene	16	0.2
1,3-Butadiene	2.25	0.08
Carbon monoxide	10.0	0.2
Nitrogen dioxide	40	13
Particles (PM$_{10}$)	40	18
Sulfur dioxide	125	2.6

asthma symptoms. However, the balance of evidence is against this hypothesis. For example, although urbanization is associated with asthma in developing countries, this is not so in developed countries, where people living in rural or semi-rural areas are equally affected. Interestingly, countries with the lowest prevalence of asthma have strikingly high levels of pollutants, including particulate matter and sulfur dioxide. In contrast, New Zealand, a country with the lowest levels of air pollution has one of the highest levels of asthma prevalence. The same is true for the Isle of Wight, a small island off the south coast of the UK. Its environment is semi-rural and the air is relatively clean, as seen by its low pollution level compared with the national air quality standard (see Table 2.2), and yet the prevalence of asthma is high.

An interesting study from Germany negated the concept that higher air pollution means more asthma. Before unification, East Germany, with its highly polluted industrialized environment, had much less asthma compared with the industrialized, but high-tech and much less polluted, West Germany. Following unification, as East Germany developed into a modern, less-polluted economy, the prevalence of asthma rose to equal that of West Germany. These studies make it difficult to blame air pollution for the rise in asthma levels in recent times.

 Fact!

The effect of air pollution on the development of asthma is small when adjusted for other factors.

Although evidence that pollution actually causes asthma is lacking, this does not mean that pollution is not important for asthma. There is plenty of evidence that individuals with asthma are very sensitive to the effect of pollutants. Experimentally, asthmatics become wheezy and develop cough at much lower level of exposure to pollutants, such as ozone or sulfur dioxide, than non-asthmatics. Exposure to outdoor pollutants in people with respiratory disease, including asthma, is a recognized cause of morbidity and mortality. The outdoor air pollutants primarily originate from exhaust fumes and particulate matter due to combustion of fuel or from industry (see box below). Particulate matter is the term used to describe tiny particles (such as carbon) present in the air, which, because of their small size, can be inhaled into the lung and reach the small airways, where they irritate the lining and cause inflammation. Exposure to pollution is an important cause of asthma exacerbation. The effect of viral infection, which is the most common cause of asthma exacerbation, is also increased in the presence of high levels of pollution. A recent study has shown that the hospital admissions for asthma increase by 1% for every 10 µg/m3 increase in small-sized particles (less than 10 µm diameter).

Common pollutants

- Ozone (O_3)

- Sulfur dioxide (SO_2)

- Nitrogen dioxide (NO_2)

- Carbon dioxide (CO_2)

- Carbon monoxide (CO)

- Methane (CH_4)

- Particulate matter

- Benzene

- Tobacco smoke

- Formaldehyde

- Volatile organic compounds

Fact!

Pollutants can interact with allergens and viruses to increase each other's effect on asthma and cause asthma exacerbation.

Within buildings, there are many items, appliances, and activities that emit air pollutants. However, the distinction between outdoor and indoor air pollutants is not clear, because some air pollutants in buildings come from outdoors. Many outdoor pollutants do not remain airborne when they enter buildings because they become attached to indoor surfaces from which they may or may not later be released. Potentially, indoor air pollutants can greatly exceed outdoor levels. It is important that people with asthma consider this when they seek to use their homes or other buildings as refuge from the effects of outdoor pollution. The impact of indoor emissions on air quality depends directly on ventilation and air mixing. Traditionally, ventilation rates have been set at levels sufficient to prevent stuffiness and odours for occupants, not to remove indoor emissions. This practice, together with recent efforts to conserve energy, has led to a situation in developed countries where the rate of exchange of indoor and outdoor air has been reduced, particularly in colder climates. Under such conditions, even low emission rates in houses can result in concentrations of indoor pollutants at levels of concern.

In summary:

- in addition to heredity, the environment in which the child grows up influences the risk of asthma development;

- interaction between the individuals' genes and the environment, especially in early life, eventually determines whether someone will develop asthma;

- it is likely that genes are important for some aspects of asthma and the environment for other aspects, and that together they cause the condition to develop;

- once a person has developed asthma, environmental exposure to allergens, pollution, and infections continues to triggers the symptoms and cause exacerbation.

Why is asthma more common in developed countries?

These findings raise the possibility that it is the Western way of living, rather than pollution, that has something to do with the development of asthma.

Various theories have been put across to explain the wide variation in the prevalence of allergic diseases. One of the most interesting theories is the 'hygiene hypothesis'. This theory proposes that childhood infections are necessary for normal development of the immune system. A limited number of infections was considered 'normal' a few decades ago. However, our obsession with cleanliness and hygiene has led to a reduction in the number of infections children get, resulting in a lack of this essential stimulant for development of the immune system. This results in a deviation in the developing immune system towards an excessive response to allergens, culminating in allergic sensitization, and asthma and rhinitis. There are several pieces of evidence supporting this hypothesis, as follows.

1. Due to improvements in public health measures including vaccines, childhood infections such as hepatitis A, measles, etc. have become much less common.

2. Allergy occurs less often in children from large families. The explanation offered is that children in large families tend to acquire more infections (from each other), and are therefore less likely to develop asthma and allergy.

3. The same reason is given for the fact that children who attend daycare centres have fewer allergies.

4. Children brought up in a farm environment have less allergic disease, possibly due to their high level of exposure to bacterial products found in the farm environment.

Thus, the rising prevalence of atopy and the falling incidence of childhood infections may be linked. However, this cannot be the whole explanation, because certain infections can increase the risk of asthma.

Other theories have suggested a variety of possible causes (see box overleaf). The widespread abandonment of breastfeeding that occurred in the 1950s and 1960s in the West was thought to expose children to cows' milk allergens early in life. Our indoor environment also changed with increased use of central heating, and well-insulated, carpeted houses led to increased exposure to house dust mite allergen. This increased exposure to food and dust mite allergen may have caused increased allergen sensitization and asthma. There is much evidence to support this theory, but some studies have failed to find a direct link between increased allergen exposure and asthma. Another possible explanation is a change in our diet over the last few decades, including less consumption of vitamins (such as vitamins E and C) and oily fish. Another theory is that increased use of antibiotics in infancy and loss of essential nutrients from our food due to modern farming methods may have resulted in a significant change in the balance of the bacteria that populate our gut. These are known to be important for healthy digestion and immune function, and this change may be a reason for the increase in allergy. Although there are various theories and arguments to explain the increase in the prevalence of allergic diseases, it should be remembered that none has been proved beyond doubt.

Proposed theories for the increase in allergy prevalence

- The 'hygiene hypothesis'
  - Increased cleanliness
  - Increased use of antibiotics
  - Increased vaccination
  - Less natural exposure to bacterial products
- Allergen exposure
  - Use of cows' milk formula
  - Increased house dust mite allergen exposure
- Dietary changes
  - Reduction in the amount of breastfeeding
  - Lack of antioxidants in the diet (vitamins C and E)
  - Lack of vitamin D
  - Lack of oily fish (omega-3 fatty acids)
  - Lack of organic food
  - Changes in intestinal (healthy) bacteria
  - Use of pasteurized milk

Evolution of asthma from childhood to adulthood

Wheezing occurs commonly in early childhood, but often this is transient and, in two out of three children, it improves or disappears. This transient wheezing in young children is generally due to viral infections or exposure to parental cigarette smoke rather than allergy and does not develop into asthma. However, in some children, wheezing persists and these are the children often diagnosed as having asthma. Parents often ask if their wheezy child will become asthmatic. There is no definitive test, but wheezy children with severe wheezing needing hospital admission, and those with a family history of asthma and children shown to be sensitized to allergens by a skin test are at much higher risk of persistent wheezing and asthma.

There is another round of asthma remission that occurs during adolescence. At least 50% of children with asthma become symptom-free as young adults, but in some, asthma comes back in later life. Severe asthma, allergic tendencies, being female, and having a family history of asthma indicate an increased likelihood of persistence of asthma through adolescence. Thus, asthma is more common in boys, but less common in men. We do not know the reason for this gender reversal, but it may be related to obesity and the fat deposition that occurs in women around puberty. Clearly, asthma and wheezing during childhood are complex entities, presenting with different characteristics at different ages. Genetic factors are clearly important, but environmental factors operating at different developmental stages also appear to influence the development of asthma.

3

How asthma affects us

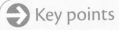 Key points

- In asthma, the single most important abnormality is inflammation of the airways (breathing tubes)

- This inflammation results in narrowing of the airways, which causes asthma symptoms

- Appropriate treatment can revert the airways back to a healthy state

- Untreated inflammation over a period of years causes permanent damage

Asthma is a disease of the airways. Airways are breathing tubes that carry air from the nose to the lungs and back from the lungs to the nose. Any problem in the airways means that air cannot be delivered to the lungs, which in turn means a reduction in the availability of oxygen to the body for important and vital functions. The patency of the airways and their normal functioning is therefore of utmost important to the overall preservation of our health.

To understand what happens in asthma, it is important to be familiar with some basic facts about the airways and lungs, and their normal function. We can then try to understand what happens to the airways and lungs in people with asthma, how it affects the normal function, and what can be done to improve the structure and function of airways to restore normality.

The following are some facts about breathing.

- All living organisms, including plants, animals, and bacteria, 'breathe' or respire.

- Breathing is an essential function that provides oxygen to the body.

- Oxygen provides energy that keeps us all alive.

- The way in which different living organisms 'breathe' is hugely different.

- Humans breathe through the nose to take oxygen into the lungs.

- When we breathe out, we get rid of the 'by-product' of the body work, a gas called carbon dioxide (CO_2).

- Carbon dioxide is exhaled with every breath and is blown out of the lungs.

The lungs are specially structured to perform these functions in an efficient and uninterrupted manner. In the next section, we will look at this in a bit more detail.

Structure of the lung and airways

The chest contains two lungs, one on the right and one on the left side of the chest. Each lung is made up of sections called lobes. The right lung has three lobes (upper, middle, and lower lobes), whilst the left lung has two (upper and lower) lobes. The lung is soft or spongy and is protected by the ribcage. When fresh air is breathed in through the nose and/or the mouth, air travels down the trachea or 'windpipe'—this is the tube in the middle of the chest and can be felt through the skin at the front of the neck. Behind the trachea is the oesophagus or 'food tube'. When we inhale, air moves down the trachea and when we eat, food moves down the oesophagus (gullet). The path taken by air and food is controlled by a structure in the throat called the epiglottis, which works as a flap that prevents food from entering the trachea. Occasionally, food or liquid may enter the trachea by mistake (i.e. it goes down the 'wrong way'), resulting in choking and coughing.

The trachea divides into a left and right breathing tube, and these are termed bronchi (Figure 3.1). The left bronchus leads to the left lung and the right bronchus to the right lung. These breathing tubes continue to divide into a complex system of smaller and smaller tubes. This is called the bronchial tree, with the following major divisions:

- trachea;

- main bronchus (to the right and left lung);

- lobar bronchus (to each lobe);

- segmental bronchi (to each segment of the lobes);

- small bronchi (several levels);

- bronchioles;

- terminal bronchioles.

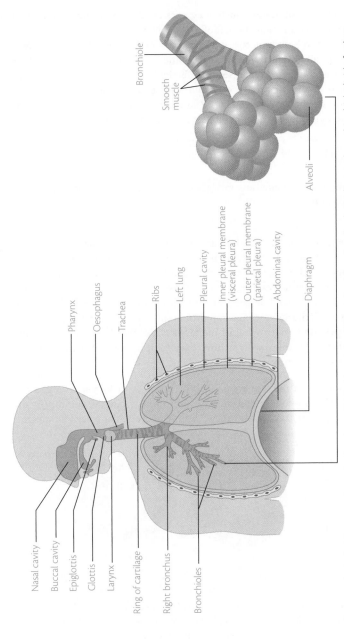

Figure 3.1 There are two lungs in the chest, divided into lobes. The main airway (trachea) divides into bronchi, which divide further, ending in alveoli.

The terminal bronchioles end in tiny air sacs called alveoli through alveolar ducts. Alveoli, which means 'bunch of grapes' in Italian, look like clusters of grapes attached to breathing tubes. There are over 300 million alveoli in normal lungs. Not all alveoli are in use at one time, so the lung has many to spare in the event of damage from disease, infection, or surgery. The alveoli, the working parts of the lung, have very thin walls that are full of blood vessels. The walls are so thin that oxygen in the air can pass through them to enter the bloodstream and travel to cells in all parts of the body.

 Fact!

If the alveoli were opened up and laid out flat, they would cover the area of a tennis court.

The trachea and bronchi are circular tubes that carry the air to the alveoli. The structure is partly hard (made up of cartilage) and partly soft (made up of membrane), and the structure circles around the tube. Inside this circle is a band of smooth muscles (Figure 3.2). When the lungs are irritated, these muscle bands can tighten, making the breathing tube narrower as the airways try to keep the irritants out. The rapid tightening of these muscles is called a bronchospasm, i.e. narrowing of the airways. A bronchospasm may cause serious problems for those with asthma, because it is more difficult to breathe through narrowed airways.

The inner surface of the airways is lined by a thin layer known as a mucous membrane. The mucous membrane is continuous from the larynx (in the throat) above to the trachea and throughout the bronchial tree. The mucous

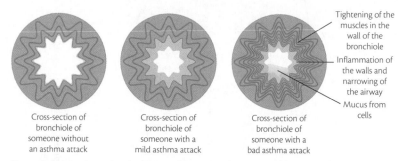

Cross-section of bronchiole of someone without an asthma attack

Cross-section of bronchiole of someone with a mild asthma attack

Cross-section of bronchiole of someone with a bad asthma attack

Tightening of the muscles in the wall of the bronchiole

Inflammation of the walls and narrowing of the airway

Mucus from cells

Figure 3.2 In asthmatics, the lining of the airway becomes congested with thick secretions leading to airflow obstruction. This is compounded by the muscles around the airways, which constrict when there is an asthma attack.

membrane is composed of sheets of cells, among which are those that secrete mucous. This mucus is 'swept up' toward the mouth by little hairs called cilia that line the breathing tubes. Cilia move mucus from the lungs upward towards the throat to the epiglottis, where it is mostly swallowed.

 Fact!

An average of 3 ounces of mucus is secreted onto the lining of the breathing tubes every day.

How do we breathe?

Like most body functions, breathing is controlled by the brain. The amount of oxygen required by the body determines the level of breathing. The breathing centre in the brain constantly receives signals from the body about the amount of oxygen that is required. The intensity of this signal will depend on the level of activity. When we are asleep, the demand for oxygen is less, and therefore breathing is relatively slow and shallow. When we are running or exercising, the demand for oxygen from the body, especially the exercising muscles, is high. These muscles send signals to the brain asking for more oxygen. Once the brain knows how much oxygen is needed, it sends messages along nerves to the breathing muscles so that the right amount of air is breathed into the lungs.

Many different muscles are used in breathing. These include:

- the diaphragm (a large muscle that lies between chest and abdomen);
- muscles between the ribs;
- scalene muscles (muscles in the neck);
- abdominal muscles.

When the diaphragm moves down or flattens, the ribs flare outward, the lungs expand, and air is drawn in. This process of breathing in is called inspiration or inhalation. When the diaphragm relaxes, air leaves the lungs and the ribs spring back to their original position. This breathing out is called exhalation or expiration. The lungs, like balloons, require effort and energy to inflate, but no energy is needed to get the air out.

What happens in asthma?

In asthma, the airways are narrowed, resulting in difficulty in air getting in and out of the lung. When the airways are narrowed in this way, there is increased resistance to breathing (the same as trying to breathe through a narrow straw). This makes it hard to get air in and out of the lungs, producing the symptoms of asthma. These include a sensation of breathlessness or breathing difficulty, partly due to the increase work of breathing as asthmatics try to force the air through the narrow passages using extra muscular strength of the diaphragm, the ribs muscles, and the abdominal muscles. The air rushing through the narrow passages also produces the whistling sounds called wheezing. Thus, the main symptoms of asthma—breathlessness and wheezing—are due to narrowing of the airways. This narrowing is the result of:

- tightening of the muscles around the airways causing bronchospasm;

- swelling of the inner lining or mucous membrane causing further narrowing of the airways;

- increased production of mucous, which is thick and blocks the lumen even further.

These three changes are the result of airway inflammation. Although it has been known for nearly fifty years that asthma is associated with inflammation of the lining of the airways, the importance of this inflammation was not fully appreciated until the 1980s. Since then, it has been established that inflammation is the primary abnormality in asthma and that everything else follows as a result of this. This notion has been further supported by the fact that inflammation was demonstrated even in subjects with very mild asthma who rarely had symptoms and did not often require any treatment. Thus, if you have asthma, you have inflammation of the airways. An expert panel that got together in 1995 thus defined asthma as an inflammatory condition (see box).

Definition of asthma

Asthma is defined as a chronic inflammatory disease of the airways characterized by recurrent episodes of wheezing, breathlessness, chest tightness, and coughing, particularly at night or in the early mornings. These episodes are usually associated with widespread, but variable, airflow obstruction that is reversible either spontaneously or with treatment.

The definition highlights two important points: firstly, that inflammation of the airways is the basic abnormality that causes asthma symptoms; and secondly, that the narrowing that occurs as a result of this inflammation can improve, sometimes on its own, but certainly with treatment.

What is inflammation?

Inflammation is the body's response to injury, infection, or irritation. Inflammation takes various forms. Sunburn is a type of inflammation of the skin in reaction to the ultraviolet rays of the sun, whilst the rash of poison ivy is another kind of inflammation of the skin, an allergic reaction to oils in the leaves of poison ivy. If someone has an injury, this is associated with swelling, redness, pain, and heat at the site of injury. In asthma, the inflammation is in the inner lining of the airways or the bronchi, but like a poison ivy rash or sunburn, the treatment is based on reducing the inflammation and preventing any further irritation to the airways.

Inflammation in asthma

In asthma, inflammation is often produced as a result of an allergic reaction occurring in the lining (mucosa) of the airways. When children with a genetic tendency for asthma and allergy are exposed to allergens, they produce a particular type of antibody called immunoglobulin E (IgE). These antibodies are primed to react to that specific allergen (Figure 3.3). When an asthmatic subject is re-exposed to the same allergen, these antibodies react with the allergen causing a series of events that occur on the surface of the airway lining or mucosa as follows.

1. The small blood vessels in the mucosa dilate, causing increased blood circulation.

2. The minute pores in the walls of the blood vessels become larger.

3. Water, cells, and proteins pour out of the blood vessels into the mucosa, causing swelling and engorgement of the mucosa.

4. Once out in the mucosa, the blood cells become activated.

5. These inflammatory cells release their contents containing a number of chemicals (known as mediators, because they mediate inflammation).

6. These mediators stimulate glands in the mucosa to produce increased amounts of thick mucous.

7. The mediators also stimulate the bronchial muscles to contract, causing constriction and narrowing of the bronchial tubes.

As a result of this inflammatory process, the asthmatic subjects develop breathlessness and wheezing (due to narrowing of the air passages). The excess

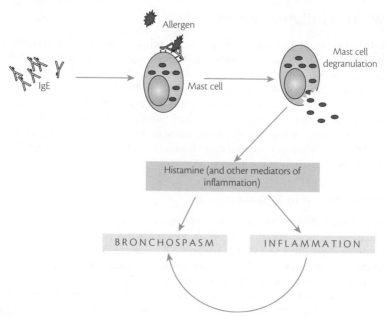

Figure 3.3 Airway inflammation in asthma. Exposure to a triggering allergen leads to release of substances by the cells in the airways, which can lead to inflammation and narrowing of the airways.

amount of mucous in the airways irritates the mucosa and initiates the coughing mechanism to get rid of the excess mucous. The sputum (phlegm) that is produced is often thick and tenacious, and comes out with difficulty. The presence of inflammatory cells in the mucous makes the airway lining irritable and twitchy, and thus ready to react to everyday irritants, such as smoke or dust, with contraction of the airway muscle, causing further narrowing. This state of irritability is often termed as 'bronchial hyper-responsiveness'.

This whole process is self-perpetuating, so that mediators cause more cells to come out of the blood vessels and these cells secrete more mediators, resulting in chronic (or persistent) inflammation. There are mechanisms in the body that try to suppress and control this excessive inflammatory response of the airway. After isolated episodes of allergen exposure (for example, an asthmatic who is allergic to cats making a short visit to a house with cats), airway inflammation is usually contained. In other words, if the exposure is short and limited, the body's own controlling mechanisms may be enough to overcome the inflammation. However, with recurrent or continuous inhalation of allergens, such as occurs with house dust mite, it is not difficult to imagine how the inflammatory response continues unabated and requires medical intervention, in the form of anti-inflammatory treatment.

 Fact!

The airways of asthmatics are sensitized to various agents. These act like triggering factors to precipitate an asthma attack.

Characteristics and consequences of asthma inflammation according to severity

Mild (intermittent/persistent) asthma

As stated above, a key discovery was that some inflammation is present in the bronchial tubes of people with asthma, even when their asthma is mild, they feel well, and their breathing is normal. The inflammation may be so mild that it does not cause significant narrowing of the bronchial tubes (Table 3.1). However, it is the underlying minimal, but persistent, inflammation that makes the bronchial tubes 'twitchy' or vulnerable to a variety of stimuli in the world around us, whether it is dust, exercise, cat dander, or cold air.

Table 3.1 Features of mild asthma

Status	Consequence
Minimal persistent inflammation	Mild cough and phlegm may occur
Mild twitchiness of the airways	Exposure to irritants, such as smoke and dust, might cause cough and wheezing
Occasional bronchial narrowing	Occasional wheezing (usually on exposure to allergens, or as a result of viral infections or exercise)
Peak flow may show some variation	Occasional need for rescue (blue) inhaler
Usually, normal lung function	Good exercise capability
Rarely get an exacerbation	Good quality of life

Table 3.2 Features of moderate asthma (if untreated)

Status	Consequence
Persistent inflammation	Cough and phlegm occurs regularly
Moderate twitchiness of the airways	At risk of symptoms on exposure to irritants
Bronchial narrowing occurs regularly	May cause regular wheeze and/or chest tightness
Peak flow shows variation, such as morning drop	Nocturnal and/or early morning cough/wheeze require rescue (blue) inhaler
Lung function—some abnormality is common	May affect exercise capability
Intermittent exacerbation, which may be moderate or severe	May affect quality of life

Moderate asthma

Most people have either mild or moderate asthma. Those with moderate asthma make up the bulk of people requiring active and regular treatment. It is in this group that preventive treatment makes a huge difference to asthma control (Table 3.2). If left untreated, uncontrolled airway inflammation may lead to frequent symptoms, significant twitchiness, and long-term complications, whereas preventive treatment with adequate control of inflammation results in few symptoms and good lung function.

Table 3.3 Features of severe asthma

Status	Consequence
Persistent severe inflammation	Cough and phlegm occur regularly (despite treatment)
Severe twitchiness of the airways	Airways react even to low-level exposure to irritants
Bronchial narrowing occurs regularly and frequently (despite treatment)	Symptoms of wheeze and chest tightness occur on a daily basis; need rescue (blue) inhaler
Peak flow shows large variations indicating instability of airways	Nocturnal and/or early morning wheezing
Abnormal lung function	Exercise limitations
Frequent and severe exacerbation	Poor quality of life

Severe asthma

A small group of asthmatics (about 5% of all asthmatics) do not respond adequately to standard treatment. They tend to have some symptoms and abnormal lung function despite treatment (Table 3.3). They also have persistent inflammation of the airways, which requires treatment with high doses of inhaled and/or oral steroids. Oral steroid treatment is associated with significant side effects. However, if this inflammation is left untreated or is inadequately treated over a period of years, the airways become scarred with permanent narrowing of the airways (irreversible damage).

Summary

In summary, our breathing apparatus is divided into a bronchial tree (breathing tubes), which leads to millions of air sacs or alveoli (the soft tissue of the lung). The breathing mechanism is very efficient with lots of spare capacity. In asthma, it is the bronchial tree that is affected by inflammation. This causes narrowing of the airways, making it difficult to breathe. Adequate treatment reverses and normalizes these changes.

4

Assessment of asthma

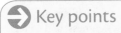 Key points

- Asthma diagnosis is usually easy, but a series of tests may help to make the diagnosis in difficult cases

- Spirometry is the single most important lung function test for the diagnosis and management of asthma

- Allergy skin prick tests help to identify relevant allergens

- The ability to monitor nitric oxide in exhaled air may prove useful in guiding the need for anti-inflammatory treatment

The first step in caring for asthma is to make a confident and correct diagnosis, and the second is to assess its severity. Only then can appropriate treatment be prescribed, and further monitoring and treatment adjustments should result in good control of asthma with few long-term complications.

Usually, it is not difficult to make a diagnosis of asthma. However, the symptoms of asthma can occur with other chest and heart conditions, and occasionally it does present a problem. There is no single test that can, on its own, be used to confirm or refute the diagnosis of asthma. Initially, typical symptoms would make one consider the possibility of asthma. A clinical history is therefore the first step, followed by physical examination and then a series of laboratory tests to reach a final diagnosis, at which point a severity level can be assigned.

Clinical history

The four most common symptoms of asthma are:

* cough (with or without phlegm);

* wheeze or whistle;

* chest tightness;

* difficulty breathing.

An asthmatic subject can present with any one or a combination of the four main symptoms. Some people present with cough and nothing else (cough-variant asthma), some describe wheezing as the only symptom, whilst others may have a combination of cough and wheezing or cough and chest tightness, and so on.

When taking the clinical history, three main categories of information are obtained.

1. *Type and frequency of symptoms.* This information helps to grade the severity. Asthma is a highly variable disease. Thus, asthmatic subjects do not have symptoms all of the time (except those with severe asthma). Those with mild, intermittent asthma may only have symptoms occasionally, i.e. on exposure to an allergen or irritant. Others may only get symptoms during viral infections. Subjects with moderate asthma have frequent symptoms and thus require regular treatment. Symptoms often occur at night or worsen at night, awakening the patient.

2. *Any exacerbating and relieving factors.* This question aims to seek information that might help avoidance. Due to the allergic nature of asthma, many different triggers make asthma worse, including allergens of different kinds, pollutants, and infection.

3. *Effect on daily life.* Specific questions on how much asthma has affected the patient's daily life help to establish the relevance of asthma symptoms in the patients' lives and the need for treatment. For children, it is important to know whether they have lost any school days and whether they are able to participate in physical activities. Similarly, assessment of severity cannot be completed without knowing whether the asthma has affected work or leisure activities. It is also useful to know about associated allergic conditions (such as eczema or rhinitis), because they may also affect the quality of life.

Children under the age of 5 are a special case. Cough and wheezing can be noticed, but they do not complain about chest tightness or difficulty breathing.

Indeed, they may simply present as having a reduced level of activity, being lethargic, and no longer wishing to play physical games. Until rapid breathing, wheezing, and coughing becomes obvious, the condition of many children with asthma may go undetected. A trial of asthma medications can help with diagnosis in some children. In very small children, the diagnosis is often confused with chest infections, which also present with wheezing due to the small size of the breathing tubes at this age.

Physical examination

A doctor or trained nurse can listen to the chest with a stethoscope for signs of asthma. This examination may reveal wheezing that is not otherwise obvious. It may also tell us how difficult it is for the air to get into the chest (and get out), and how much air is going in and out. It may tell us about any infection that might be present. Finally, it helps to exclude other conditions that might be confused with asthma. However, in asthma, a physical examination may be completely normal. A repeat examination following treatment can be useful. The airway obstruction is considered reversible if the wheezing disappears in response to treatment, or when the suspected triggering factor is removed or resolved.

 Fact!

With narrower breathing tubes in asthma, it is usually more difficult to breathe out, which means a longer time is needed to breathe out compared with breathing in.

Investigations

Investigations are carried out for diagnosis, to assess severity, and to monitor control of asthma. Investigations focus on:

◆ measuring lung function;

◆ identifying allergies;

◆ assessing and monitoring (recent) airway inflammation.

Blood tests are not particularly helpful in the management of stable asthma (they are helpful in managing an asthma attack). A chest X-ray is usually done only if there is suspicion of chest infection or of an alternative diagnosis.

During an asthma attack, a blood test may indicate the possibility of infection and thus the requirement for antibiotics. Examination of the level of oxygen in the body is important. This can be done with a probe attached to the finger tip. For a more comprehensive assessment of the level of gases (oxygen and carbon dioxide) in the body, a small sample of blood may be required. This also provides an indication of the severity of the attack and whether breathing support in an intensive care unit may be needed. A chest X-ray is done in most instances to exclude infections or other complications.

Lung function tests

A major abnormality in asthma is narrowing of the airways causing obstruction to airflow. The degree of this obstruction can be assessed using lung function tests. There are several types of lung function test or pulmonary function test. Spirometry is one of the most useful tests and can be performed

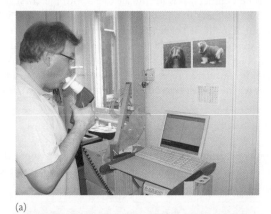

(a)

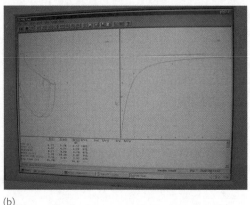

(b)

Figure 4.1 Use of a spirometer (a) and the resultant output chart (b).

easily in an office setting, using a piece of equipment called a spirometer (Figure 4.1a). This is a simple test and takes only 2–3 minutes to perform. The procedure involves blowing hard into the spirometer. After taking a deep breath, the person breathes out into the spirometer, as completely and forcefully as possible. The spirometer measures both the amount of air expelled (volume) and how quickly the air was expelled from the lungs (flow). These measurements are recorded by the spirometer (Figure 4.1b).

There are three major types of information we can get from this procedure: firstly, the total volume of air that was blown out; secondly, the volume of air blown out in the first second; and thirdly, the maximum speed with which the air is blown out (Table 4.1). These three parameters are essential to make an objective assessment of asthma. They tell us about slightly different aspects of lung function and together they give a good assessment of how lung function is affected in asthma. The forced vital capacity (FVC) measures the overall volume of air and is reduced in asthma, as well as in many other chest conditions. The forced expiratory volume in 1 second (FEV_1), on the other hand, is more closely related to the width of the bronchial tubes. With normal-width tubes, around 80% of the air comes out in the first second, but with asthma, where the bronchial tubes are narrowed, this is significantly reduced.

 Fact!

We can normally breath out in the first second (FEV_1) approximately 80% of the total volume of air that we are able to blow out (FVC). Only 20% comes out in the remaining 3–4 seconds.

Table 4.1 Volumes and flow obtained from spirometry that are commonly used to diagnose and monitor asthma

Parameter	Explanation
Forced vital capacity (FVC)	This measures the total amount of air one can blow out, with force, after as deep an inhalation as possible. The total time it generally takes for someone to breathe out fully is around 4–5 seconds, but may be longer in asthma.
Forced expiratory volume in 1 second (FEV_1)	This measures the maximum amount of air one can blow out in the first second.
Peak expiratory flow (PEF)	This is the maximum flow achieved during a forceful blow out. This reading tells us how quickly the air can be blown out of the lungs.

Thus, although both FEV_1 and FVC are reduced in asthma, FEV_1 is reduced more than FVC and hence the ratio of FEV_1 to FVC is reduced. This ratio (called the forced expiratory ratio), which is normally around 0.8 (depending on age), is the most reliable indication of the degree of narrowing of the bronchial tubes (airflow obstruction) and therefore a low forced expiratory ratio is called an obstructive defect. If an obstructive defect is demonstrated by spirometry, in the right clinical setting, this would be highly suggestive of a diagnosis of asthma.

Spirometry is a safe test. Sometimes mild coughing and wheezing can be caused by repeated vigorous attempts at forceful breathing. This usually clears rapidly on its own, but occasionally may require a couple of puffs of a reliever inhaler (bronchodilator).

In relation to spirometry, there are three other points to be considered:

- what is normal and what is low?

- variation in spirometry;

- reversibility.

Normal values

Like any other test, normal values are derived from averages of a large number of healthy people. A range of values are regarded as normal, although healthy values change from person to person, depending on:

- age;

- height;

- gender;

- ethnicity.

Tables have been created to indicate normal values for a person based on age, height, gender, and ethnicity. An asthmatic subject's spirometry values are compared with those that would be expected and then assigned a percentage. For example, a person with asthma may have an FEV1 that is 70% of the expected or predicted value. Because there is some normal variation and not everyone has a value of exactly 100%, anything above 85% of the predicted value is considered normal.

Fact!

Spirometry values are affected by age, height, gender, and ethnicity, but not weight!

Variation

Asthma is a highly variable disease. Asthmatic patients may feel well one day and ill the next, depending on a variety of factors and exposures. Although an obstructive defect (a low forced expiratory ratio) on spirometry is highly suggestive of asthma, if spirometry is done on a good day and it is normal, this does not exclude a diagnosis of asthma. Mild asthmatics may have normal lung function most of the time, whereas most severe asthmatics do show some abnormality all of the time. However, even in these, spirometry can vary widely. This variation can occur on its own (spontaneous) or with treatment; the latter is called reversibility. Significant spontaneous variation in spirometry, without an obvious alternative cause, is almost always diagnostic of asthma. Alternatively, an improvement with treatment can be sought to make a diagnosis in difficult cases.

Reversibility

Reversibility can be tested using a bronchodilator (i.e. a drug that opens the airways in the lungs) or steroids. Bronchodilators act quickly and therefore it is easier to demonstrate bronchodilator reversibility. Spirometry is first performed (as a baseline). The patient then inhales a bronchodilator and the spirometry is repeated. If the values of the test performed after administration of the bronchodilator are significantly better than the pre-bronchodilator values, then the obstruction is considered reversible. Sometimes a patient with asthma does not demonstrate reversibility after inhalation of a bronchodilator. In this situation, the patient may be treated for a few weeks with steroids to improve his or her underlying airway inflammation and then return for a repeat spirometry test. If the post-treatment spirometry results are significantly better than the initial results, the obstruction is considered reversible.

 Fact!

A improvement in spirometry results, either spontaneously or following treatment, is a cornerstone of the diagnosis of asthma.

Case study

Overbreathing in asthma

A 30-year-old receptionist was referred to the asthma clinic with a history of worsening asthma control. Three years previously, her family doctor diagnosed asthma and, during this period, her asthma treatment had to be increased repeatedly due to poor control. She had at least six exacerbations during the previous 12 months, requiring oral steroids. On questioning, her main symptom was difficulty in breathing. There were no irritants or allergens in the environment, and she did take her inhalers and medications as prescribed. On examination, she appeared anxious, but a chest examination and chest X-ray were normal. However, specialized breathing tests indicated that, although her lung functions were normal, she was overbreathing, causing a sense of breathlessness (a condition called hyperventilation syndrome). This occurs due to excess anxiety, which may not be obvious. She was reassured and, following breathing exercises by a physiotherapist, it was possible gradually to reduce her treatment level to a low-dose preventer inhaler taken twice a day. Despite this planned and supervised reduction in her treatment, her asthma control remained good.

Peak expiratory flow

Because asthma symptoms vary, it is not unusual for a patient with chronic asthma to have normal spirometry results. In such cases, monitoring of peak expiratory flow (PEF) rate may be used to diagnose asthma. PEF is a reading that is obtained during spirometry (the maximum flow achieved). However, the same reading can also be obtained with a peak flow meter, which is a portable, inexpensive, hand-held device (Figure 4.2). This measures air flow from

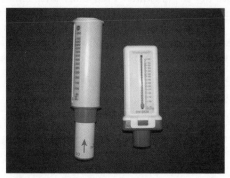

Figure 4.2 Peak expiratory flow meters.

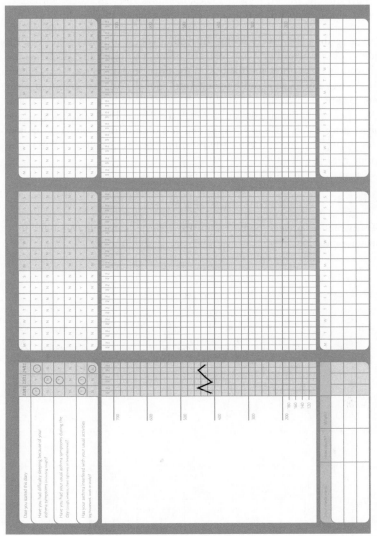

Figure 4.3 Example of a peak flow diary. Reproduced with the kind permission of Asthma UK© Asthma UK 2008.

the lungs and records the maximum flow. The meter has a marker that slides up the scale as the person blows out. In simple terms, this measures how hard and quickly one can push air out of the lungs. PEF readings are measured in litres per minute. In normal individuals, the lungs and airways are normal, so they are able to blow out better and hence get a higher PEF reading.

A single reading is not very useful. Instead, it is best to take a series of PEF readings over a period of a few weeks at home. The individual performs the PEF reading three times and the best of the three readings is recorded (Figure 4.3). A common error is not blowing hard enough. Another common error is not putting the lips right around the mouthpiece to create a good seal and make sure that all the air goes out through the device. PEF readings are done at least twice a day, once in the morning and once in the evening. Peak flow varies during the day and the early morning peak is usually lower than the evening peak (Figure 4.4).

 Fact!

A variability of greater than 20% in PEF indicates sufficient variability to diagnose asthma.

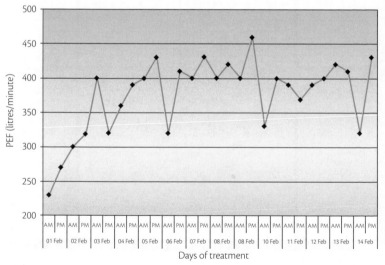

Figure 4.4 Variability of PEF in an asthmatic patient characterized by dips in lung function.

To take a PEF reading, one should use the following procedure.

1. Check that the pointer is at zero.

2. Preferably stand in a comfortable, upright position.

3. Hold the peak flow meter level (horizontally) and keep the fingers away from the pointer.

4. Take a deep breath and close your lips firmly around the mouthpiece to create a good seal (Figure 4.5).

5. Blow as hard as you can—as if blowing out candles on a birthday cake. It is the speed of blow that is being measured, not the amount of air blown out.

6. Look at the pointer and check the reading.

7. Reset the pointer back to zero.

8. Repeat this three times and record the highest reading in the asthma diary card.

A peak flow meter can be used by most adults and children over 6 years of age. PEF readings vary according to the age, height, and sex of a person. PEF values can also vary from person to person, and the doctor or asthma nurse can provide advice on one's best PEF.

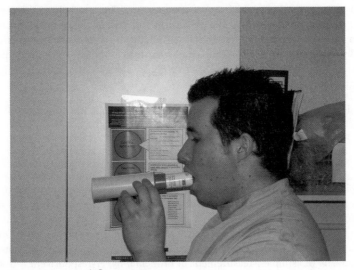

Figure 4.5 Using a peak flow meter.

In people with diagnosed asthma, PEF monitoring can provide useful information regarding asthma control. PEF readings are done at least twice a day, before any asthma medications are taken. Regular PEF monitoring may provide early warning signs of a deterioration in asthma control. Records of PEF readings provide the doctor or asthma nurse with information on asthma control and help with decisions on changes to asthma treatment. Furthermore, a PEF reading may help to identify causes of asthma at work, home, or play, and may help parents determine what might be triggering their child's asthma.

 Fact!

During an asthma attack, PEF readings can determine the severity of the problem, and help in deciding when to use the reliever inhaler and determining when to seek emergency care.

Bronchial provocation tests

In some patients with symptoms suggestive of asthma, routine spirometry and a PEF diary may not demonstrate variable or reversible airflow obstruction (Figure 4.6). In such circumstances, a test to demonstrate another characteristic of asthma, i.e. 'twitchy' airways, can be used to confirm the diagnosis. This test is called bronchial provocation testing. The idea behind this test is that stimulating the bronchi of a person with an irritant will result in constriction due to contraction of the muscles around it. If the bronchi are twitchy or easily irritable, they will constrict at a lower dose of the irritant, thus demonstrating bronchial irritability or hyper-responsiveness. Common methods used to provoke bronchial muscles are:

◆ inhalation of chemicals such as histamine, methacholine, or mannitol;

◆ physical agents, such as cold air;

◆ a natural stimulus, such as exercise.

Subjects perform spirometry at the beginning of the test. One of these methods is then used in gradually increasing amounts, while the symptoms and spirometry results are closely monitored. The dose of chemical, for example, that makes the FEV_1 decrease by 20% is noted and the test is stopped. Given an appropriate history, a demonstration of bronchial hyper-responsiveness is diagnostic of asthma. Measurement of bronchial hyper-responsiveness is also useful in assessing the severity of asthma.

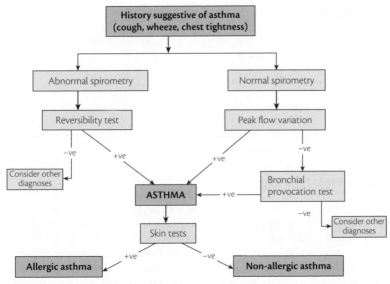

Figure 4.6 Asthma diagnosis: a flow diagram to show the tests that can be used, and in what order, to make a diagnosis of asthma if there is uncertainty. A skin test (or blood test) can be used to decided whether it is an allergic or non-allergic asthma and to identify allergens. Key: +ve, positive; −ve, negative.

 Fact!

Not all patients with asthma have bronchial hyper-responsiveness and not everyone who demonstrates bronchial hyper-responsiveness has asthma.

This test has been shown to be safe. Many patients undergoing this test do not have any symptoms at all. However, inhalation of the provoking agent may be associated with asthma symptoms in some. A bronchodilator is always administered at the end of the test to reverse the effects of the provoking agent. The test is carried out in such a way that the dangers of a severe asthmatic reaction are minimized. However, there is a small risk of precipitating severe narrowing of the airways and therefore this test is usually done in a medical setting.

Diagnosis

The diagnosis of asthma is demonstrated by cough, wheezing, and chest tightness, plus one of the following:

- variable obstruction in air flow (FEV_1 or PEF);

- reversibility using bronchodilator or steroid;

- bronchial hyper-responsiveness (deterioration following exercise or after administration of a provoking agent).

Skin prick testing

Identification and avoidance of allergens is an important part of asthma management. Allergy testing—either by skin testing or by measuring antibodies in the blood—can tell us if the asthma is allergy-induced and, if so, the specific allergens involved. Thus, skin tests helps to confirm the sensitivity to the allergenic trigger, so that appropriate avoidance advice can be provided. It is important to note that all test results must be interpreted in the context of a careful history. The common groups of allergens tested in asthma include:

- house dust mites;

- furry animals, such as cats and dogs;

- pollens, such as grasses, trees, and weeds;

- moulds, such as *Aspergillus, Candida* and *Alternaria*

The skin prick test is usually carried out on the inner forearm, but can be performed on the back. Ideally, the allergens should be selected in accordance with the patient's history. Anything from one to around thirty allergens can be tested. The skin is coded with a marker pen for the allergens to be tested. A drop of the allergen solution (extract) is placed by each code. The skin is then pricked through the drop using the tip of a small needle. This introduces a tiny amount of allergen into the skin (Figure 4.7). This can feel a little uncomfortable, but should not be painful. With a positive reaction to an allergen, the skin becomes itchy within a few minutes, and then becomes red and swollen with a 'weal' in the centre (very much like the reaction to a nettle sting). The weal has a raised edge, which slowly expands to reach its maximum size in about 15–20 minutes. The size of the weal varies, with the average being 3–5 mm in diameter, and for most people it clears within an hour. The size of the weal broadly indicates the level of sensitivity. A positive skin test to an allergen corresponds to the level of antibodies to that specific allergen in the blood.

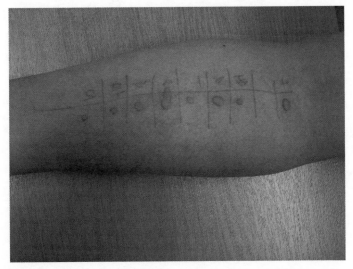

Figure 4.7 Example of a skin prick test.

 Fact!

A skin prick test is safe and almost any age group can be tested, including babies.

Exhaled nitric oxide

Nitric oxide is a gas that is produced by inflammatory cells. Because asthma is an inflammatory disorder of the airways, the level of nitric oxide is increased in exhaled breath and this can be measured. This is a simple test in which the patient breathes out into a device and the fraction of exhaled nitric oxide (FeNO) in the total air that comes out is recorded (Figure 4.8). This is similar to a breathalyser test used to measure the amount of alcohol in the blood. Those with inflammatory conditions of the airways such as asthma and rhinitis tend to produce more nitric oxide than healthy individuals and the proportion in the exhaled air is higher. This gives an indication of the degree of airways inflammation present. The results are available immediately and are helpful in guiding treatment. Treatment of airways inflammation with inhaled steroids reduces the FeNO and this is being used as a new tool to adjust the dose of inhaled steroids.

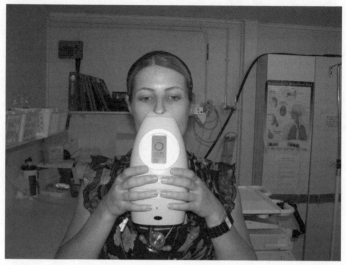

Figure 4.8 Measurement of exhaled nitric oxide for assessment of airways in asthma.

5

Allergen avoidance

 Key points

- Avoidance of a relevant allergen by an asthmatic may prevent symptoms and exacerbations and may reduce the need for medication to control the disease

- The most relevant allergens for people with asthma are those that are inhaled and are present all year round, such as house dust mites, moulds, pets, and cockroaches

- A comprehensive approach is required for reduction of house dust mite allergens and avoidance measures should be carried out over the whole house

- An important step for reduction of house dust mite, mould, and cockroach allergens is to eliminate their reservoirs and make the environment hostile to their survival

The role of the immune system is to fight off infections. However, in some people, the immune system develops in such a way that it also reacts to a few substances that are not harmful. Allergens are substances, usually proteins from plant, food, or animals, with the ability to stimulate the immune system. Exposure to these allergens can cause the immune system to overreact, leading to various symptoms, depending on the organ system involved. If the symptoms are confined to the nose/eyes, it causes the familiar hay fever or allergic rhinitis, whilst involvement of the lower airways results in asthma, and the skin is primarily affected in eczema. Occasionally, multiple organ systems are involved, when it is called systemic allergic reaction or (when life-threatening) anaphylaxis.

The idea of allergen avoidance is interesting and appealing. In theory, avoidance of a relevant allergen by an asthmatic will:

- prevent the occurrence of symptoms;

- improve disease control;

- reduce the amount of treatment required.

This strategy works for some allergens, but not for all, and in reality this can be very difficult. For example, allergens such as foods, drugs, and latex can be successfully avoided for the most part, but inadvertent exposure to food allergens is still common. However, these allergens are not the most relevant in chronic asthma. Allergens that make asthma worse are those that we inhale, such as house dust mite, mould, and cockroach allergens, and less commonly pollens. Avoidance is difficult for these allergens. Still, a reduction in exposure may be helpful in improving symptoms. The important thing is to know where these allergens are likely to be found, what indicates their presence, and what can be done to reduce exposure. A structured allergen avoidance plan and advice can help these patients to gain good control over their asthma, in addition to their medication-induced control.

 Fact!

All asthma-management guides recommend the avoidance of allergens as far as is reasonably possible.

The first step is to find out what the individual asthmatic is allergic to. This is done with either a skin prick test or a blood test (to measure antibodies specific to the allergens, i.e. specific IgE) (see Chapter 4). All asthmatics should be routinely tested against a battery of perennial (all-year-round) aeroallergens to determine their sensitivities. They may also be tested against pollens if there is a hint of seasonal components to their symptoms. Rarely, foods are suspected triggers, in which case these may be added to the list of allergens to be tested.

 Fact!

Not all patients have allergic asthma. Studies have shown that up to 30% of children and 40% of adults may have non-allergic or non-atopic asthma.

Following a skin prick test, those who are found not to have allergic asthma, i.e. whose skin prick test is negative to common and relevant allergens, can be reassured that they do not need to worry about allergen avoidance. Those who are found to be allergic following a skin prick test can be given appropriate advice on allergen avoidance. However, simply having a positive result against an allergen in a skin prick or blood test is not sufficient reason to start undertaking expensive and time-consuming avoidance measures. The relevance of the allergy to patients' symptoms also needs to be established. This is achieved by taking a detailed and comprehensive history. For example, a person found to be allergic to house dust mites and pollen following a skin prick test, but with only seasonal symptoms (pollen asthma) need not take measures to reduce dust mite exposure.

Aeroallergens

Aeroallergens are airborne substances, such as pollens or fungal spores, that can cause allergic disease. The most important indoor allergens are house dust mites and cockroaches, whilst outdoor allergens are grass, trees, and weed pollens. Fungal spores and allergens of animal origin can be found both indoors and outdoors.

House dust mites

House dust mites (or dust mites) are invertebrates with eight legs (Figure 5.1) and belong to the same group as spiders and scorpions (class Arachnids).

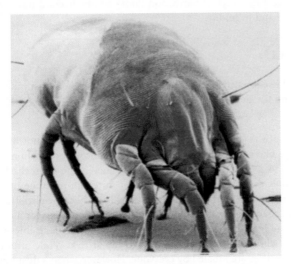

Figure 5.1 A house dust mite. Magnification ~2000×.

However, they are very small and not visible unless viewed under a micro-scope. They like similar temperature and humidity conditions to humans. They have a life span of 2–3 months and can survive at temperatures of 15–35°C and, ideally, high humidity levels (75–80%). They do not drink water but absorb moisture from the environment. We are the providers of their food. Humans continually shed skin and lose about 6 grams of dead skin each week. Dust mites feed on this as well as on animal dander and other biological mate-rials in the dust, such as pollen and fungi.

 Fact!

House dust mites live closely with us because we provide them with a place to live (such as a mattress), food (our shed skin), and the right indoor temperature and humidity conditions.

Dust mites are very good scavengers. When food is scarce, they eat their own droppings as recycled nourishment. Thus, dust mites are efficient survivors. Dust mites like to live in dark, damp, warm, and poorly ventilated areas, and consequently thrive in mattresses, pillows, soft furniture, soft toys, and thick carpets, because these materials have minute spaces, deep in the fabric pores, that provide the appropriate living conditions. Because they also feed on ani-mal dander, they will be plentiful in areas where family pets sleep. Dust mites cannot survive on vinyl or hardwood floors or under conditions of extreme temperature and humidity.

 Fact!

A typical used mattress can have 100,000 to 10 million dust mites inside, feeding on the dead skin that we shed.

Dust mites are essentially harmless to us because they do not bite or cause skin disease like scabies mites. However, a significant proportion of humans are allergic to them. The allergens they produce come from the body parts of dead mites and their droppings. A dust mite can produce up to twenty droppings a day. These particles are very small and become airborne when the dust is disturbed. For example, every time someone walks over a carpet, mite dust is spread into the air and will take two hours to settle. Babies and young children crawling on the carpet are especially at risk. While airborne, these allergenic particles are inhaled by everyone. However, when a dust mite-allergic patient is exposed to them, they will develop symptoms of asthma, a runny nose, or eczema. There is strong scientific evidence that dust mite allergy is causally related to asthma. The evidence includes the following.

- It has been observed that communities with high amounts of dust mite allergen tend to have more asthma in both adults and children.

- It is believed that 75–85% of allergic asthmatics are sensitized to dust mites.

- Experimental inhalation of small doses of dust mite allergen in people with mild asthma reproduces asthma-like symptoms and at higher doses may cause an asthma attack.

- Drastic measures, such as removing children to an environment free of dust mites (such as an alpine resort high in the Alps), can have a dramatic effect on reducing asthma symptoms.

- Asthmatics with dust mite allergy consistently improve, over a few months, when kept in a mite-free environment in a hospital.

Thus, it is generally accepted that dust mite allergen avoidance can be a useful adjunct in the management of dust mite-sensitive asthmatic patients. In infants at high risk of asthma, controlling the levels of dust mite allergen may prevent the development of asthma in some children. However, it is not easy to get rid of these creatures or to reduce allergen exposure significantly. Isolated measures, such as applying mattress covers only, do not work. A more comprehensive approach is required and, for the best results, the avoidance steps should be carried out throughout the whole house. The three aims of a dust mite reduction programme are as follows.

1. To eliminate dust mite reservoirs, e.g. by removing carpets.

2. To kill dust mites, e.g. by hot washing of bedding etc., and by reducing indoor humidity.

3. To put a barrier between the dust mites and humans, such as mite-impermeable bed covers.

It may take at least two months before the effects of carrying such avoidance measures are noticed. To reduce exposure to dust mites in the house, the following recommendations are useful:

- wash or dry-clean pillows and bedcovers regularly, at 56°C or higher, if possible;

- leave bedcovers turned back during the day;

◆ leave windows open where and when it is sensible to do so;

◆ avoid drying clothes indoors, especially in the bedroom and living room, unless using driers that are vented outdoors. If you have to dry clothes indoors, open a window and close the door to the room where the damp clothes are;

◆ vacuum mattresses, carpets, upholstery, etc. thoroughly every two weeks;

◆ dispose of, and replace, mattresses and pillows over ten years old;

◆ steam-wash carpets on a regular basis;

◆ if possible, get rid of carpets. It is difficult to clean wall-to-wall carpets thoroughly, even with steaming;

◆ replace carpets with sanded and varnished floorboards, or a vinyl, linoleum, tiled, or purpose-made wooden floor. Use a minimum of scatter rugs and wash these several times a year. In cold climates, hanging the rugs outdoors in freezing weather helps;

◆ dust mite-allergic patients should damp-dust instead of vacuuming;

◆ replace soft cloth-upholstered furniture with dust-proof furniture;

◆ adding a mite-killing substance in a low-temperature wash can kill mites in bedcovers and other washable items that will not stand a high-temperature wash. Benzyl benzoate is an important ingredient;

◆ dehumidifiers can be useful to reduce the dampness in a house;

◆ encase mattress, pillows, and duvets in mite allergen-impermeable covers and regularly launder all uncovered items, preferably at 60°C;

◆ do not give furry toys to children to take to bed.

Cockroaches

Cockroach sensitivity is an important cause of asthma in the USA and in some other parts of the world with warmer climates, although it is a less likely trigger in the UK. These creatures, present in many homes, are a major cause of year-round indoor allergies. In the USA, cockroach infestation is a problem among households in inner cities or in the south, in particular in those of low socioeconomic background. Cockroach allergy is more common among African Americans. Experts believe that this is not because of racial differences, but because of the disproportionate number of African Americans living in inner cities. In one study of inner-city children, 37% were allergic to cockroaches, 35% to dust mites, and 23% to cats. Those who were allergic to cockroaches and were exposed to the insects were hospitalized for asthma three times more often than other children.

 Fact!

It is believed that well over three-quarters of urban homes in the USA have cockroaches. Each infested home may house 800–300,000 cockroaches.

When one cockroach is seen in the basement or kitchen, it is safe to assume that at least 800 cockroaches are hidden under the kitchen sink, in closets, and elsewhere. The allergens from cockroaches come from the insects' faeces, saliva, and bodies. Cockroaches are one of the most resilient organisms and can survive extreme conditions. However, prevention of exposure to these allergens is usually successful if appropriate measures are applied. It has been shown that if these interventions are maintained, then cockroach allergen levels will decrease in the house within 12–24 months. The preventive measures include the following.

- Remove food sources and household food wastes. Foods should be stored in sealed containers.

- Do not leave out pet food or dirty food bowls.

- Reduce access of the cockroaches to water. Fix leaking taps and/or prevent water condensation on pipes.

- Improve ventilation to eliminate damp areas.

- Caulking or sealing cockroach access and entry points helps, including repair of cracks and holes in wall.

- Spray cockroach runways around kitchen cabinets and drawers with insecticides known to kill cockroaches. Insecticides will kill the parent cockroach, but will not kill their eggs. Therefore, repeated spraying every 1–2 months is necessary for effective control of cockroach populations.

- Thorough and frequent housecleaning is required to remove dust and cockroach by-products.

Animal dander

There are an estimated 13 million cats and dogs in the UK. In the USA, more than 70% of households have a dog or cat. Pets provide companionship, security, and a sense of comfort. However, up to 10% of the UK population may be allergic to pet animals to some degree, and for those with asthma this rises to almost 30%. Dander (old skin scales, similar to, but much smaller than, dandruff on the human scalp) is the major source of pet allergens and is constantly shed into the environment. These allergens are extremely tiny, like a dust or powder, and allergy sufferers seldom, if ever, know they are circulating in the air, clinging to furniture, curtains, wall coverings, etc. If a dog or cat has been in the family for a long time, its dander will have permeated the entire household. There is no relationship between how long your pet's hair is and how much dander its skin produces. However, although dog or cat fur is not a major allergen, it does collect pollen, dust, mould spores, and other irritants.

 Fact!

One of the major causes of allergic reactions to dogs and cats is not their hair or fur, but dander, which is dried skin scales.

Dander occurs naturally as the outer layer of skin (epidermis) renews itself. The epidermis of dogs and cats is quite thin; it is made up of many layers of cells that are constantly pushing outwards to replace the cells above. This outer (superficial) layer of cells dies and flakes off into the environment as dander. In addition to dander, there are other sources of allergens from cats, dogs, and other animal in frequent contact with humans (Table 5.1). In dogs, saliva and urine are also potential sources of allergens. They are deposited on the fur through licking and urination. Dogs often scratch themselves, which facilitates removal of the allergens from the skin and fur to be spread around. Also, when the hair dries, the microscopic particles on its surface flake off, become airborne, and trigger the symptoms that characterize allergies to pets. Cats produce other major allergens, present in the secretions of the glands of the skin and in saliva. This allergen is deposited on the fur from skin gland secretions and through saliva when cats lick themselves clean. Again, when these allergen particles dry, they become airborne. These cat allergens are particularly sticky and can be carried on clothing to environments that do not have cats, such as schools. A cat allergy is more common than a dog allergy.

With rabbits, rats, mice, hamsters, and guinea pigs, the most important sources of allergens are the saliva and urine. Once dry, these secretions become airborne, and can be a source of allergic reactions for children and laboratory animal workers.

Table 5.1 Major sources of allergens from animals

Animal	Source of allergen
Cat	Dander, skin gland secretions, saliva
Dog	Dander, saliva, urine
Rabbits, rats, mice, hamsters, and guinea pigs	Saliva, urine
Horse, cow	Skin scales
Budgie	Droppings

Horse and cow skin scales can be allergenic to those exposed to them. Budgie droppings can release proteins into the air that can induce asthma. Birds can also carry allergy-provoking mites, moulds, and pollen on their feathers.

People are emotionally attached to their pets and it is important to make an accurate diagnosis of a pet allergy. Skin prick tests and a blood test can help, but these tests should be interpreted with the background information available following a comprehensive history. For example, do the patient's symptoms improve when he or she is away from the pet's environment for a week or two, for example, when on holiday? If a pet allergy has been confirmed, complete avoidance is the best recommendation, so the pet should be found another home.

 Fact!

Pet allergens may remain in the home for up to six months after removal of the pet.

If the family or allergic person is unwilling to remove the pet, the following advice is useful to reduce the amount of allergens in the household.

- The family should avoid replacing their furry pets when they die.

- The pet should at least be kept out of the patient's bedroom and, if possible, outdoors. Indoor pets should be restricted to as few rooms in the home as possible.

- Allergic individuals should not pet, hug, or kiss their pets because of the allergens on the animal's fur and saliva.

- The pet should be kept off any furniture in a room where the person spends most of their time, because exposure can be very high.

◆ Litter boxes should be placed in an area unconnected to the air supply for the rest of the home and should be avoided by allergic individuals.

◆ The allergic person should always wear a protective mask and gloves when grooming the pet.

◆ Clothing worn after grooming or playing with pets should be removed and the clothing, now full of animal dander, kept out of the bedroom. Clothing should be washed with a washing agent that removes allergens, e.g. Allergen Wash.

◆ The pet should be washed regularly—allergens can easily be washed away with a wet sponge (wearing gloves when washing the pet or, better still, geting someone else to do it).

◆ Bedding with which pets have been in contact regularly should be replaced—it can take months or even years to remove allergens from fabrics.

◆ Air currents from forced-air heating and air conditioning will spread allergens throughout the house. Homes with forced-air heating and/or air-conditioning may be fitted with a central air cleaner, or a room air purifier can be used for at least four hours a day

◆ Using a high-efficiency particulate air (HEPA) vacuum cleaner or high-efficiency vacuum cleaner bags can reduce the amount of dust, allergens, and pollen pumped back into the air by the vacuum cleaner.

◆ People allergic to birds should not use feather pillows or down duvets. If a feather pillow is used, it should be encased in a protective cover, so that none of the feathers can escape.

◆ When visiting the home of a pet owner, an allergic person should request that they do not vacuum immediately before the visit because the pet allergens can remain airborne for up to a day making the allergens more likely to be breathed in.

Moulds

The term mould is synonymous with fungi. Moulds are small (microscopic) fungi. Mould particles and spores are not visible without a microscope, but they are found both indoors and outdoors. The level of exposure can be assessed by sampling the air in the relevant environment. High levels of humidity facilitate the growth of moulds and promote the dispersion of spores. Spore counts typically rise with rainfall and fog, and with damp conditions.

Moulds can survive in humidity conditions ranging from 0 to 100%, but flourish in the 65–85% range. Most allergenic moulds release their spores into the atmosphere during dry conditions (humidity below 70%); however, some prefer an environment with a high humidity for spore release.

Moulds are found in:

- damp, dark places, like cellars, bathrooms, garages, and attics;

- on rotting leaves or vegetation;

- on indoor plants and organic plant containers, such as straw and hemp;

- old foam-rubber pillows and peeling wallpaper;

- furniture stuffed with decaying cotton;

- rubber gaskets on old refrigerator doors;

- dishwashers, drainage sinks, and washing machines;

- rubbish bins;

- water-damaged areas, such as leaky roofs, walls with dry rot, and wet carpets;

- gardens and backyards with poorly maintained landscaping and large amounts of organic debris near the house, like ivy, compost, and bark chips; mould growth in these places correlates with the indoor mould spore levels, due to outside air moving in;

- room-air humidifiers, cold-mist vaporizers, and air-conditioning systems, which can significantly contaminate indoor air.

Mould allergen-induced asthma can occur in both children and adults. Mould allergies are usually perennial, but there may be significant seasonal variations that influence the level of symptoms. The degree of seasonal variation in exposure may depend on the geographical location of the patient. A large number of moulds can potentially cause allergies in humans.

 Fact!

Approximately one in four patients with allergic asthma or rhinitis is sensitized to common moulds, such as *Aspergillus*, *Cladosporium*, and *Alternaria*.

Allergen avoidance can play a key role in alleviating symptoms in patients with a mould allergy as follows.

- Avoid carpets in areas that are likely to get wet and damp.

- Use an exhaust fan or open the window to remove moisture after showers and in the kitchen when cooking, to remove water vapours to prevent moisture and damp.

- Use a dehumidifier or air conditioner to maintain humidity at less than 50%; this may be useful if the house is located in a humid environment.

- An air cleaner with a HEPA filter may help to remove floating mould spores indoors.

- Wash window sills with an anti-fungal agent to discourage mould growth.

- When first turning on home or car air conditioners, leave the windows in the room or vehicle open for several minutes to allow mould spores to disperse.

- Avoid storing unnecessary items in basements or attics where mould can accumulate.

- Regularly check pipes or duct works for leaks.

- Eliminate dense vegetation around the house.

- Avoid raking leaves, moving lawns, working with hay or dead wood, or other activities that are likely to stir up mould spores.

- Remove decaying vegetation from the roof, gutters, and garden.

- Wear a mask for outdoor work, if necessary.

Pollen

Pollen is seasonal and is a well-known cause of hay fever. Many people with hay fever have asthma and nearly 70% of individuals with asthma have hay fever symptoms. In the UK, tree pollen tends to cause symptoms early in the year, whilst grass pollen causes symptoms in mid-summer. Mould spores are usually the cause later in the year (July–November). A wet summer is more likely to lead to symptoms as a result of mould spores rather than pollen, which typically are associated with hot, dry weather.

Table 5.2 Common plants producing airborne pollens

Type of plant	Name
Grass	Timothy grass, Kentucky bluegrass, Johnson grass, Bermuda grass, redtop grass, orchard grass, sweet vernal grass
Tree	Alder, hazel, birch, horse chestnut, oak, ash, elm, hickory, pecan, box elder, mountain cedar
Weed	Ragweed, plantains, mugwort, docks

Pollen is formed from round or oval pollen grains produced by plants in order to pollinate themselves or other plants and produce seeds. Most plants want to spread their pollen over a wide area to give themselves the best opportunity for fertilization. This is called cross-pollination, i.e. in order for fertilization to take place and seeds to form, pollen must be transferred from the flower of one plant to that of another plant of the same species. The pollen is usually spread by insects or wind. Pollen causing an allergic reaction is commonly produced by trees, grasses, and weeds that do not produce showy flowers (Table 5.2).

The pollen grains of these plants are small, light, and dry, making it easy for the wind to take them up and spread them across a large area. Samples of ragweed pollen have been collected 400 miles out at sea and 2 miles high in the air. Because airborne pollen is carried for long distances, it does little good to rid an area of an offending plant (e.g. grass or tree), because the pollen can drift in from many miles away. Most allergenic pollen comes from plants that produce it in huge quantities.

 Fact!

A single ragweed plant can generate a million grains of pollen a day.

The chemical make-up of pollen is the basic factor that determines whether a particular type is likely to cause hay fever. Pine tree pollen is produced in large amounts by a common tree, which would make it a good candidate to cause an allergy. However, the chemical composition of pine pollen appears to make it less allergenic than other types. Moreover, because pine pollen tends to fall straight down and is not widely scattered, it rarely reaches the nose and airways of individuals to elicit symptoms.

Each plant has a pollinating period that is fairly constant every year. Exactly when a plant starts to pollinate seems to depend more on the relative length of night and day, and therefore on geographical location, than on the weather. The pollen count is a measure of the number of pollen grains of a certain type per cubic metre of air sampled, averaged over 24 hours. The reported counts are usually for grass and trees (in the UK) and refer to the previous 24-hour period up to 9 a.m. that day. The pollen counts show when the various seasons start and end, as well as the day-to-day variation in the amount of pollen in the air. This information can be used to take some remedial and preventive action in susceptible individuals. Pollen counts tend to be highest on warm, dry, breezy days and lowest during chilly, wet periods. Pollen concentration in an area can be influenced by:

◆ population growth;

◆ land use;

◆ tree planting and cutting;

◆ industrialization;

◆ pollution.

A pollen calendar provides information on the locally prevalent pollens for a particular month. These vary from country to country, from region to region, and within different vegetation zones. In the UK, grass pollen is the most frequent cause of hay fever, but other types are also important. Around 90% of hay fever sufferers are allergic to grass pollen and about 25% are allergic to birch pollen. In Scandinavia, birch pollen is prolific, whilst in parts of southern Spain, olive pollen ranks as the main cause of hay fever, and in North America, ragweed is an important culprit.

Some individuals who suffer from severe hay fever due to pollen allergy also get asthma symptoms, known as pollen asthma. There is a strong seasonality to their symptoms and day-to-day variation in symptoms may follow the pollen count. Avoidance of pollen is not easy and complete avoidance is almost impossible. However, those with moderately severe hay fever and pollen asthma should consider taking the following measures during the pollen season and particularly on high-pollen-count days.

◆ Avoid going outdoors during the daily peak periods of pollen exposure. These are usually between 6 and 9 a.m. when the pollen rises from the ground as the air warms up, and between 6 and 9 p.m. in the evening when the pollen comes down again as the air cools.

- Avoid drying clothes outside. Unfortunately, pollen attaches itself to the clothes in large quantities and this can produce symptoms when the washing is brought in.

- Keep bedroom windows closed, particularly during the daily peak periods, because the pollen will lie in an invisible sheet over bedroom carpets and bedding, and cause problems during the night.

- Bathe and rinse hair every night before bed to remove all traces of pollen from the body.

- Large amounts of pollen can settle in hair, so if an individual has long hair, tie it back during the day.

- Use air conditioning to reduce pollen levels by recirculating indoor air.

- Use an air-treatment system such as an electrostatic air purifier or a HEPA filter air cleaner, particularly in the bedroom.

- Keep the grass in the lawn short. Mowing should be performed by a non-allergic family member.

- Eliminate weeds by cutting them down or using a weed killer (performed by a non-allergic family member).

- Avoid direct contact with indoor and outdoor flowers.

- Wear sunglasses outside to reduce eye irritation caused by pollen.

- Consider using a filtering mask when exposure cannot be avoided.

- When driving, keep the windows closed. Use a car air conditioner with a pollen filter.

- Plan holidays when the pollen levels are high to areas where the offending pollens are less prevalent.

- Avoid unpaved parking areas and construction sites.

6

Treatment of asthma

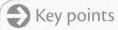

> ## Key points
>
> - With modern asthma treatments, the vast majority of asthma patients can enjoy an excellent quality of life with minimal side effects
>
> - Inhaled steroids, as preventer inhalers, are the first line of treatment for asthma and they need to be taken regularly
>
> - Reliever inhalers are used for breakthrough symptoms and are used as and when required
>
> - It is important to take asthma medicines properly, so that every dose provides the most benefit

Goals of asthma therapy

Once the diagnosis is confirmed, it is important to treat asthma effectively. The goals of asthma therapy include:

- gaining adequate control of asthma symptoms during day and night;

- maintaining normal activity levels;

- prevention of asthma attacks;

- trying to achieve near-normal lung function;

- no or minimal side effects due to the medications.

Drugs and devices used for asthma

There are excellent medicines available to help control asthma and, in the vast majority of patients, it should be possible to achieve the goals described above. Asthma is a chronic inflammatory disease of the airways and hence treatment of this inflammation is the cornerstone of asthma treatment. In addition to this, treatment is required to prevent or treat the main consequences of this inflammation. Prominent among these aims is to ensure that the bronchial tubes remain wide, so that breathing is easy and without effort. This can often be achieved with anti-inflammatory treatment alone, but additional medications are sometimes also required. If the bronchi do constrict in response to exposure to allergens or irritants, then this can quickly be reversed by drugs called bronchodilators.

 Fact!

In addition to drug treatment, measures should also be taken to avoid allergens and other triggering agents, such as smoke, pollution, sprays, etc.

Thus, there are two main types of asthma medication:

1. anti-inflammatory treatment;

2. bronchodilators.

The main anti-inflammatory medication used for the treatment of asthma is steroids. These are effective in suppressing inflammation and are very useful drugs. However, they do have side effects and attempts should be made to minimize these as far as possible whilst using the drug to good effect. The side effects of steroids depend on the dose used and how long they are administered for. If the dose is small enough, it can be used continuously, without significant side effects. This is achieved by using steroids in inhalers. Because the drug is inhaled directly into the lungs where it works locally, only a small dose is required for good effect. This type of inhaler is also called a preventer inhaler, because it prevents asthma symptoms and exacerbations due to the medication (steroids) it contains. For treatment of exacerbation, steroids are given as tablets and the dose is large. However, if the treatment is limited to a few days and not repeated often, then the side effects of the steroids are again minimal and tolerable. Some severe asthmatics need steroids continuously in large doses and these people are at risk of long-term adverse effects.

> **Fact!**
>
> Steroids are extremely useful drugs and, when used appropriately, can be
> used to derive maximum benefit with minimal side effects.

The same principal of local drug delivery to the lungs is utilized for the other
main group of asthma medications—bronchodilators. These drugs are also
taken via an inhaler and used either regularly for continuous effect (long-acting
bronchodilators) or whenever needed (short-acting bronchodilators); the latter is also called a reliever inhaler. A slight disadvantage of inhalers is that
some effort is required for effective use and that the dose delivered with one
puff is relatively small. In an exacerbation, when large doses are needed by a
patient who is breathless, it may not be possible to inhale the required dose
effectively. In these situations, a piece of equipment called a nebulizer is used
to deliver the bronchodilator (and occasionally steroids) in a mist form. Thus,
asthma treatment can be delivered by any of the following means.

- Inhalers:
  - reliever inhalers;
  - preventive inhalers;
  - long-acting bronchodilator inhalers.
- Tablets:
  - leukotriene modifiers, e.g. montelukast;
  - theophylline;
  - steroids.
- Nebulizers
- Injections

Each of these is discussed in more detail below.

Inhalers for asthma

Inhalers (also called puffers) are small, hand-held, portable devices that deliver
medication directly to the lungs (Figure 6.1). They enable children and adults

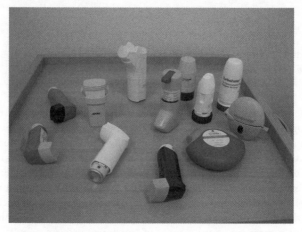

Figure 6.1 Some examples of inhalers.

with asthma to inhale medicine, almost anytime and anywhere. Inhalers have transformed asthma treatment.

> **❗ Fact!**
>
> Inhalers enable people with asthma to lead active lives without fear of an attack. This is because inhalers are portable and convenient, and can provide immediate relief.

A variety of inhalers are available to help relieve or control asthma symptoms. Two common types include metered-dose inhalers and dry-powder inhalers.

Metered-dose inhalers

These use a chemical propellant to push the medication out of the inhaler. The medication may be released by squeezing the canister or by direct inhalation. Squeezing the top of the canister converts the medication into a fine mist. Some metered-dose inhalers are activated by the act of deep breathing and do not require the person to squeeze the inhaler. The lips are placed on or near the inhaler's mouthpiece to inhale the mist (Figure 6.2). It is important to use inhalers properly in order for the medications to

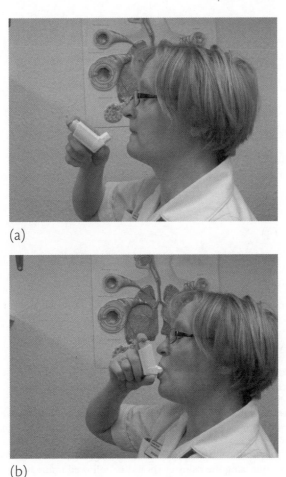

(a)

(b)

Figure 6.2 Using a metered-dose inhaler. (1) Remove the cap and hold the inhaler upright. (2) Shake the inhaler. (3) Tilt the head back slightly and breathe out, then put mouthpiece in the mouth while starting to take a breathe in, which should be slow and deep. (4) Press down on the inhaler to release the medicine and gently continue to breathe in slowly for 3–5 seconds. (5) Hold the breath for ten seconds, or as long as you can, to allow the medicine to go deep into the lungs. (6) Repeat this precedure as directed. Wait one minute between puffs—this allows the second puff to get into the lungs more effectively.

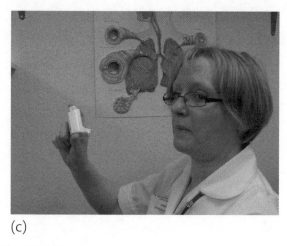

(c)

Figure 6.2 (*continued*)

be effective. The advantages of using the medication in inhaler form include that:

- the medicine works more quickly;

- the medicine is delivered where it is required, i.e. to the lungs; therefore, less medicine is needed, which means fewer side effects;

- some recent inhaler medicines are broken down after they have had their effect in the lungs, further reducing the risk of harmful side effects.

A slight problem in using a metered-dose inhaler is the need for coordinating two actions: squeezing the canister should be followed immediately by inhalation of the medication (hand–lung coordination). If the coordination is not perfect, some of the drug may escape into the air and/or be deposited at the back of the throat. People who have difficulty using this type of inhaler may find it easier to do it with a spacer. The spacer is a short tube that attaches to the inhaler (Figure 6.3). The top of the canister is then squeezed to release the drug into the spacer. The spacer acts as a holding chamber that keeps the medication from escaping into the air. Releasing the medication into the chamber gives the person time to inhale it at their own pace. This has two advantages: it decreases the amount of medicine that is deposited on the back of the throat (resulting in less throat irritation and infection) and it increases the amount of

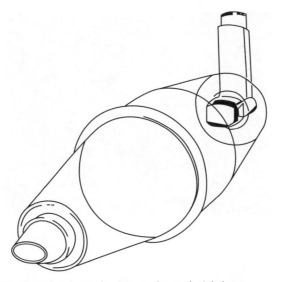

Figure 6.3 The spacer is a short tube that attaches to the inhaler.

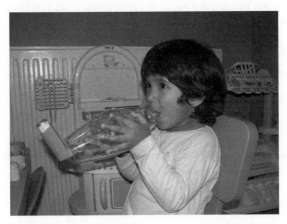

Figure 6.4 Spacers are used for young children in whom hand–lung coordination can be difficult.

medicine that reaches the lungs (improved effectiveness). Spacers are useful for young children in whom hand–lung coordination can be difficult (Figure 6.4). For infants, a mask is attached to the end of the spacer's mouthpiece. When the drug is released into the spacer from the other end, it fills the air within the spacer and is breathed in by the infant (Figure 6.5).

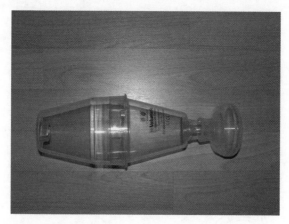

Figure 6.5 A spacer attached to a mask.

Dry-powder inhalers

These do not use a chemical propellant to push the medication out of the inhaler. Instead, the medication is released by inhaling rapidly through the dry-powder inhaler (Figure 6.6). Available types include:

- dry-powder tube inhalers (Figure 6.6);

- dry-powder disk inhalers (Figure 6.7);

- single-dose dry-powder disk inhalers.

Spacers cannot be used with dry-powder inhalers. Some patients find dry-powder inhalers easier to use than the metered-dose inhalers because hand–lung coordination is not required. However, others may not have the breathing effort required to inhale the medication into the lungs.

Reliever inhalers

Reliever inhalers, as the name suggests, relieve symptoms and are used on an 'as required' basis to ease symptoms of breathlessness and wheezing. Reliever inhalers contain drug called bronchodilators, which dilate (widen) the bronchi (airways). The dilation of the bronchi achieved by the reliever inhaler is by relaxation of the muscles around it. This makes the airways become wider and the asthmatic symptoms quickly resolve. However, the effect of a reliever

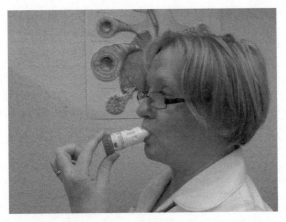

Figure 6.6 Using a dry-powder inhaler (turbohaler). (1) Breathe out. (2) Form a good seal around the mouthpiece of the inhaler device. (3) Inhale rapidly and deeply. (4) Hold the breath for ten seconds or as long as possible for the medicine to reach the deeper parts of the lungs. Try to avoid accidentally breathing out (blowing) into the device, because this can scatter the medicine.

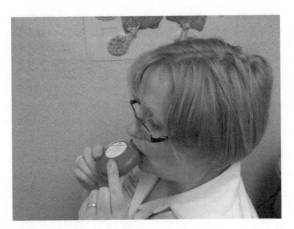

Figure 6.7 A dry-powder disc inhaler.

inhaler is transient, lasting only a few hours. Unless the trigger is removed and/or the underlying inflammation is treated appropriately, airway narrowing may recur every few hours.

> ### Fact!
>
> Reliever inhalers do not have any effect on airway inflammation, which is the main reason behind airway narrowing.

There are a number of different bronchodilators, such as salbutamol and terbutaline. These are available in various brands, made by different companies. There are different inhaler devices that deliver the same or similar reliever drugs, which thus have similar side-effect profiles (Table 6.1). The reliever drugs tend to be used in blue or grey inhaler devices. For those with very mild asthma who do not have frequent or regular symptoms, the occasional use of a reliever inhaler may be all that is required. However, if an asthmatic individual needs a reliever three times a week or more to ease symptoms, a preventer inhaler is advised.

Preventer inhalers

The mainstay of asthma treatment is the use of preventer inhalers. These 'anti-inflammatory' medications help to control swelling in the airways associated with asthma. As the name suggests, preventers are used to prevent symptoms and are thus taken daily whether asthma symptoms occur or not. The specific medication and dose are usually determined by the doctor or asthma nurse, depending on the frequency and severity of asthma symptoms. They do not provide immediate relief of symptoms and it takes a few weeks of consistent use for their effect to be felt. This is why some asthmatics give up their use

Table 6.1 Common drugs used in reliever inhalers and their side effects

Drugs	Side effects
Generic names: salbutamol, terbutaline Common brand names: Airomir, Asmasal clickhaler, Bricanyl, Salamol Easi-Breathe, Ventodisks, Ventolin	Fine shakes, headache, muscle tension, racing heart, sleep disturbance, muscle cramps, occasional fall in blood pressure

after a few days, thinking that they are not benefiting from this inhaler, and rely instead on a reliever inhaler, which gives immediate relief—they feel better, but the relief is only transient and the underlying cause of the disease is not dealt with by the reliever inhaler. Another common mistake is for asthmatics to stop using their preventer inhaler once they have improved and have few or no symptoms—their asthma gradually worsens again and the need for the reliever inhaler increases, and this can result in a serious, uncontrolled asthma attack.

 Fact!

It is a good principle that preventive medication should never be stopped without prior agreement with your doctor, even in the complete absence of symptoms.

Steroids are the most widely used medication in preventer inhalers because it has been found that steroids reduce swelling in the airways and long-term use can reverse the swelling of the airways. They are the most effective anti-inflammatory drug available and are considered to be essential for moderate to severe asthmatics. Steroid inhalers are very safe and are usually taken in doses of under 1000 micrograms (1 milligram) per day. At high dose, or if taken incorrectly, the steroid deposition in the throat can be considerable, causing fungal infections of the throat and oesophagus (gullet or feeding tube). In children, there is also some concern regarding their effect on growth. However, most studies have shown that doses below 1 milligram are safe, and even above 1 milligram, the growth-suppressive effect is transient. In other words, asthmatic children taking inhaled steroids may sometimes lag behind their peers in height gain, but eventual height is generally the same. Some of the steroids used in preventer inhalers, their common brand names and the side effects of this group of drugs are given in Table 6.2. Most of the local side effects such as oral thrush, hoarse voice, and sore throat can be avoided by gargling, rinsing, and spitting after each dose, and by using a spacer with the inhaler.

It may take up to 14 days for the preventer medication to reduce the swelling and mucus in the airways, and the full effect may not be achieved for up to six weeks. Over a period of time, the chest tightness, wheezing, and night-time cough are reduced. Once effective control of asthma is achieved, it may be possible to reduce the dose without losing control. However, it is important not to reduce the dose oneself (unless clear instructions have been provided by a doctor or nurse), because this can lead to an asthma attack. Dose adjustment is

Table 6.2 Inhaled steroids: common preparations used in preventer inhalers and their side effects

Drugs	Side effects
Steroids	
Generic names: beclomethasone, budesonide, fluticasone, mometasone, ciclesonide	Oral thrush, hoarseness of voice, anxiety, sleep disturbance, growth restriction in children, thinning of bones
Common brand names: Alvesco, Asmanex, AeroBec Forte, Asmabec Clickhaler, Beclazone Easi-Breathe, Becloforte, Becodisks, Becotide, Pulmicort, Qvar, Seretide	
Non-steroids	
Generic names: sodium cromoglicate, nedocromil sodium	Cough, throat irritation
Common brand names: Cromogen Easi-Breathe, Intal, Tilade	

generally done under the guidance of a doctor or an asthma-specialist nurse. Once protection is working and the asthma is stable, occasionally forgetting the dose should not compromise the control of the asthma.

 Fact!

Regular omission of the dose, stopping the preventer medication for several days at a time, or using the inhaler randomly or infrequently means that the protective effect of the medication will disappear and asthma symptoms will recur.

Only a tiny minority of preventer inhalers use medication that is not a steroid (Table 6.2). These treat inflammation, just like steroids, but are not as effective (although very safe). These are used to treat mild asthma, especially in children. They are also useful in the treatment of exercise-induced asthma. Their use has gone down in recent years due to the proven safety of steroids in inhaled form, especially if the dose is kept below 1 milligram a day. Several new drugs are being researched to be used in inhaled form for preventive treatment of asthma. These are not steroids, but aim to be as effective.

Long-acting bronchodilators

In addition to reliever and prevented inhalers, there are other treatments for asthma given through inhalers. One of the most commonly used is the long-acting reliever inhaler. These drugs work on the same principal as the reliever inhaler, i.e. they relax smooth muscles around the bronchi to dilate bronchial tubes and are therefore called bronchodilators. Because their effect lasts for 12 hours (the reliever inhaler's effect lasts for only six hours), they are called long-acting bronchodilators. These include:

- salmeterol (brand name: Serevent);

- formoterol (brand names: Foradil and Oxis).

These are available both in metered-dose form and in dry-powder form. They are usually used twice a day to keep the airway muscles relaxed. Formoterol acts quickly and therefore can be used for immediate symptom control as well as the reliever effect. The side effects of long-acting bronchodilators are similar to the reliever inhalers (see Table 6.1).

 Fact!

Long-acting bronchodilator drugs have little or no effect on inflammation in the airways. They should always be used in conjunction with steroid inhalers.

If asthma is not adequately controlled with a preventer inhaler alone, then a long-acting bronchodilator inhaler is added to the treatment (Figure 6.8). The two inhalers can be used one after another or the two drugs (steroid and long-acting bronchodilator) can be put in the same inhaler (combination inhaler). The use of combination inhalers has significantly improved asthma management. Because both of these medications are taken twice a day, this combination helps the patient by only needing to use one inhaler, but getting the advantage of two medications, thereby optimizing the asthma treatment.

Oral medication (tablets)

If inhalers are not sufficient to manage the disease, add-on treatments for asthma are available as tablets.

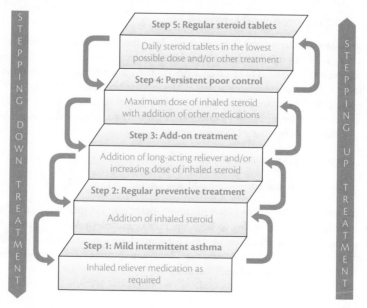

Figure 6.8 Stepwise management of asthma.

Leukotriene modifiers

These are one of the newer preventive medicines. They can be used alone or in combination with inhaled steroids. However, they are commonly used if additional treatment is required after inhaled steroids and long-acting bronchodilators (Figure 6.8). These act like steroids, i.e. they suppress inflammation, but they are not steroids and therefore do not have the side effects of steroids. Again, they are not as effective as steroids and should not be used routinely in place of inhaled steroids. They are useful as a supplementary therapy, before other treatments are considered that may cause more side effects (such as theophylline or steroid tablets).

Leukotrienes are a type of chemical in the body that contribute to the airway inflammation of asthma. This type of medicine interferes with the effect of leukotrienes in the body, either by stopping leukotrienes from being made or by blocking their action. This helps to reduce and prevent swelling inside the airways. It also stops mucus from forming and reduces muscle tightening around the airways. Leukotriene modifiers are usually taken in the evenings. This group of medicines should not be used as relievers in an acute asthma attack because they are not effective in this situation. They are generally well tolerated, but do have some side effects (Table 6.3).

Table 6.3 Commonly used leukotriene modifier drugs

Drug	Side effects
Generic name: montelukast Brand name: Singulair	Abdominal pain, thirst, headache, diarrhoea, nausea, abnormal dreams, joint pains, fatigue itchiness, rash
Generic name: zafirlukast Brand name: Accolate	Headache, skin reactions, fatigue, sleeplessness, joint and muscle pains, liver function abnormalities

Theophylline

This drug is used in a small group of asthmatics who do not respond to the more commonly used treatments described above (Figure 6.8). The drug has a unique ability to reduce airway inflammation (preventer effect) and also open up the airways (bronchodilation reliever effect). This is a time-tested medication that has been in use for four to five decades. However, its side-effect profile is generally worse than other asthma medications (Table 6.4). The occurrence of these side effects is related to the levels of the drug in the blood and it is recommended that the dose is adjusted to keep the blood levels within a narrow range, so that it is effective, but not toxic. This requires monitoring by blood tests, which is inconvenient.

Oral steroids

Like inhaled steroids, oral steroids or steroid tablets are used for the treatment of asthma. They are usually given in a short burst during an asthma flare-up or in low doses for long-term use in severe asthmatics whose symptoms are not controlled by the standard treatment (Figure 6.8). Steroid tablets work quickly and effectively to reduce the redness and swelling of the airways. Steroid tablets are very good for the control of asthma, but, because of the potential side effects, they are reserved for use only in an emergency or in very poorly controlled asthmatics. Steroid injections are sometimes used in an emergency, but their advantage over the tablet form is not proven. When oral steroids are

Table 6.4 Theophylline and related drugs

Drugs	Side effects
Generic names: theophylline, aminophylline Brand names: Nuelin SA, Slo-Phyllin, Uniphylin Continus, Phyllocontin Continus	Headache, nausea, vomiting, abdominal pain, racing heart, agitation, fits (rarely), irritability, lack of sleep

given as a short burst (for less than two weeks), it is not essential that the dose is reduced gradually before stopping it.

 Fact

Oral steroids for short bursts (duration of two weeks or less) can be started and stopped abruptly, without the need for a gradual reduction.

However, when given for longer-term use—for example, to bring asthma under control in severe asthmatics, which might take weeks or months—they should be gradually reduced and not stopped abruptly. This is because our body produces natural steroids that are essential for several important body functions. The requirement for, and the production of, natural steroids increases during periods of infection and stress. When outside steroids are used for more than three weeks, the adrenal glands, which produce natural steroids, become 'lazy' and stop making their own steroids. Thus, in the event of an infection or stress, the body cannot cope, because the required surge in steroid production is missing. This lack of steroids may cause low blood pressure, shock, and death. A person on long-term steroid treatment requires a booster of steroids in case of sudden illness or injury for any reason. They should carry an identification tag stating this fact, so that if they are become unwell enough not to be able to tell anyone, this fact can be known and steroids can be given immediately.

 Fact

If an asthmatic has been on long-term oral steroid treatment, the dose must be tapered off gradually to allow time for the adrenal glands to start functioning again.

Side effects of steroids

The worry about side effects of steroids is mainly when they are taken orally for long periods. The long-term side effects are usually in proportion to the dose and duration of treatment. A short burst of steroids is usually well tolerated. Some of the side effects that may be experienced by patients are given in Table 6.5.

Avoiding the side effects of steroids

Keeping asthma under good control will reduce exacerbations and hence the need for steroids. This is achieved by the regular use of preventer inhalers and

Table 6.5 Side effects of steroids

Treatment	Side effects
Short burst (given as hydrocortisone injections or prenisolone tablets)	• Increased appetite • Mood changes (high mood or depression) • Fluid retention • Indigestion
Long-term treatment (repeated short bursts or regular usage; usually given as prednisolone tablets once daily)	• Increased appetite and weight gain • Thinning of bones, which can lead to weak bones that may break easily • Slow-down of growth in children • Suppression of body's own production of steroids • Easy bruising of the skin and slow healing of cuts • Puffiness or roundness of the face • Indigestion or stomach ulcers • Fluid retention with swelling of the ankles • Cataracts in the eyes • Difficulty in controlling diabetes • Chicken pox can become a serious problem • Suppression of the body's defences against infection (this may result in unusual infections that can be difficult to treat)

any add-on treatments, and the avoidance of allergens and irritants. For individuals on long-term steroid tablets, the following advice is useful.

◆ Avoid smoking, because concurrent smoking can worsen the bone thinning induced by steroid tablets.

◆ Take steroids in the morning to mimic the natural production of steroids in the body.

◆ Taking calcium tablets regularly can help to strengthen bones. Specific preventative treatment to avoid bone thinning may also be necessary.

◆ Regular exercise improves bone strength.

◆ Eat sensibly to avoid putting on weight.

Nebulized medications

Nebulizers create a mist of water and asthma medicine (as a solution) that is breathed in. They can deliver more of the drug, and to exactly where it is needed, than conventional inhalers. The most commonly used medications in a nebulizer are the short-acting bronchodilator (reliever) medicines. Occasionally, steroids can also be given in this way. The medication in solution form is placed in a chamber that is connected to an air compressor, which is powered by electricity (through the mains or by a battery). The compressor blows air through the chamber, making a mist of the medication solution, so the patient can inhale it through a mouthpiece or face mask. The major advantage of this system is that it requires essentially no hand–breath coordination and very little effort from the patient. Thus, it can be used for young children, and those who are very ill and unable to cooperate. Also, a large dose can be delivered within a few minutes, so this is very useful for an acute asthma attack. This is why nebulizers are often used in hospitals or by general practitioners to treat asthma exacerbations. Occasionally, for those with severe asthma, nebulizers can be used at home, either as required or for regular use.

How to use a nebulizer

A nebulizer should be used as follows.

1. Pour the medication solution into the nebulizer cup.

2. Attach the mouthpiece or mask to the cup (a mask may be easier for young children).

3. Place the mouth around the mouthpiece or put the mask on the child's face.

4. Switch on the nebulizer.

5. If the person can follow directions (i.e. they are not too young or too ill), they should take deep, slow breaths and hold each one for 1–2 seconds before breathing out. Otherwise, the mist should be inhaled by natural breathing efforts.

6. Continue breathing until all of the medication in the cup is used up.

7. Rinse the cup and mouthpiece or mask after each use.

Injection treatment

Several asthma medications can be given by injection including steroids, bronchodilators, and theophylline and related drugs. However, this route is usually reserved for treatment of an asthma attack in hospital. Recently, a new treatment has become available for allergic asthma, which is given by injection as a regular treatment to control chronic severe asthma. This drug, called omalizumab, works by neutralizing an allergic antibody (immunoglobulin E or IgE). IgE is important for the initiation and continuation of allergic inflammation in the airways. Once the IgE has been neutralized, the allergic inflammation tends to subside, which improves asthma control. This injection is given every 2–4 weeks, depending on the level of IgE antibodies prior to treatment, to keep the IgE levels down. This treatment is, however, very expensive and not without side effects. It is thus usually reserved for severe asthma patients not responding to other treatment.

 Fact!

A new class of drug has recently become available to control severe allergic asthma and acts by neutralizing the effect of allergic antibodies.

Management of asthma

The modern management of asthma is guided by evidence-based guidelines. Typically, a stepwise approach is taken to provide optimum asthma control (Figure 6.8). First, it is important to determine the goals of treatment, and to agree realistic and achievable targets with the patient and their family.

Stepwise management of asthma

Initial treatment

An assessment of asthma severity needs to be made before the appropriate treatment level can be decided. The doctor or nurse makes a judgement as to which step the patient fits into and decides on the initiation of treatment appropriate to the severity of the asthma at the time of evaluation. If adequate control is not achieved, the treatment is gradually stepped up until good control is achieved. Alternatively, treatment can be started at a higher level from the start to achieve rapid control and then stepped down to the minimum treatment required to maintain control. A higher level of treatment can be achieved by adding a short course of steroid tablets or using a higher dose of inhaled steroids. The second approach is preferred because it provides rapid control of airway inflammation.

Stepping up

If adequate control is not achieved within 4–6 weeks, the treatment is stepped up. This procedure is repeated until adequate control is achieved. If asthma is not controlled with a reasonable amount of medication in a compliant patient, then the diagnosis should be revised or the existence of a complicating factor investigated.

Stepping up of the treatment is done whenever there is evidence of poor asthma control. This includes night-time awakening due to asthma, an urgent visit to the emergency department for an asthma attack, or increasing need for the use of rescue medications.

 Fact!

In some individuals, a short burst of steroid tablets may be required to re-establish control during a period of gradual deterioration of asthma.

Prior to increasing the asthma medications or stepping up the treatment, it is important to check the inhaler technique of the patient, to check whether inhalers are being used on a regular basis as advised, and to attempt to find out whether anything has changed in the environment or living/working conditions of the patient. Sometimes, patients do not comply with asthma treatment due to a real or perceived fear of side effects or simply due to carelessness, but they do not tell their doctor for fear of upsetting them. This may result in further, possibly unnecessary, treatment being prescribed.

Monitoring

Even when control of asthma symptoms has been achieved, increases or decreases in medication may be needed, because asthma severity and control vary over time. It is important to have follow-up visits every 3–6 months to monitor the asthma. In addition, home monitoring of peak flows is essential, because this provides objective evidence of the effectiveness of asthma control at home and at work.

Stepping down

Stepping down or reducing the medication is done gradually after several weeks or months of adequate asthma control, when the goals of treatment are being met. In general, the last medication to be added on to the treatment is the first to be reduced. Inhaled steroids can be reduced gradually, for example by 25% of the dose at a time, until the minimum dose required for good asthma control is reached. Patients with severe asthma who are treated with regular or frequent oral steroids should be seen regularly by asthma specialists. Patients should be monitored closely for side effects and constant attempts should be made to reduce the dose of steroid tablets, albeit under medical supervision.

Management of asthma in special situations

Exercise-induced asthma

A diagnosis of exercise-induced bronchospasm is suggested by a history of cough, shortness of breath, chest pain or tightness, wheezing, or endurance problems during and after vigorous activity. The diagnosis can be confirmed by an objective measure of the problem, e.g. a 15% decrease in peak flow or FEV_1 between measurements taken before and after vigorous activity. Exercise-induced asthma should not limit an individual's participation or success in vigorous activities. One of the best examples is Olympic athlete Jackie Joyner-Kersee, who suffered from asthma, but went on to win a gold medal at the 1988 Seoul Olympic Games.

Appropriate steps should be taken to reduce the risk of exercise-induced symptoms as follows.

- Try covering the mouth and nose with a scarf or a face mask if exercising outside in cold weather.

- Always breathe through the nose while working out, because this helps to warm the air that goes into the lungs.

- Warm up for 15 minutes before starting to exercise.

- Exercise is better tolerated in short bursts.

- Swimming is a preferred type of exercise because it is not likely to cause symptoms.

- Take medication prior to exercise, if needed.

The use of a reliever medication immediately prior to working out should prevent narrowing of the airways. Other medications such as a long-acting reliever or sodium cromoglicate inhaler may also be effective. Teachers and coaches should be made aware of the problem so that the individual can take the necessary medications prior to a workout. If symptoms happen with usual or regular activity, a stepping up of the treatment is recommended. If the patient continues to be symptomatic despite adequate treatment, an alternative diagnosis should be considered.

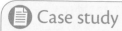 Case study

Exercise-induced asthma

A 22-year-old receptionist was seen in the clinic because she found that she was not able to do her activities at the gym. She was putting on weight, and the doctor had advised her to take some exercise and get fitter. Therefore, she started eating sensibly and joined a gym. However, she found that after ten minutes of exercise she was out of breath. She was not able to exercise for any longer than this. She had a family history of asthma, but denied any asthma symptoms or allergy. After examination, she was provided with a peak flow meter to record the readings before and after exercise. There was a significant reduction in her peak flows after exercise. She was prescribed a reliever inhaler and her symptoms improved markedly. She was able to do normal workouts in the gym and used her reliever inhaler prior to exercise. This lady had exercise-induced asthma, which was readily controlled with relievers.

Seasonal asthma

Seasonal asthma, a form of allergic asthma, can be triggered by trees, grasses, or flowers releasing pollen into the air. For example, some people find that their asthma is worse in the spring, when there is an increase in tree pollens. Others find their asthma is worse in the summer due to grass pollen, or in late summer and early autumn when ragweed and mould are more likely to cause problems. Thus, people with seasonal asthma only get asthma symptoms during the pollen season of the allergen to which they are sensitive. These patients may benefit from the following:

- avoidance of the relevant allergen;

- an increase in preventive treatment prior to the season in which they are affected;

- starting on an inhaled steroid a few weeks before the anticipated onset of symptoms. The medication should be continued throughout the season;

- adequate treatment of nasal symptoms, because this will improve asthma symptoms.

Management of asthma during pregnancy

The treatment of asthma during pregnancy is no different from treating asthma in non-pregnant women. If asthma is not well controlled during pregnancy, it can result in a reduced oxygen supply to the fetus, reduced growth, and prematurity. There is little evidence to suggest that regular asthma medication harms the foetus. Inhaled steroids alone or in combination with long-acting bronchodilator medications are the preferred choice for the management of persistent asthma. Studies and observations of hundreds of pregnant women with asthma have demonstrated that most inhaled asthma medications are appropriate for patients to use while pregnant. Steroid tablets are not preferred in the treatment of asthma during pregnancy. However, they can be used to treat severe asthma attacks during pregnancy. If they have to be used regularly in very severe asthmatic patients, their potential risks are still less than the possible risks of severe uncontrolled asthma.

 Fact!

The risks of uncontrolled asthma appear to be greater than the risks of necessary asthma medications.

Other aspects of asthma management need to be highlighted, including identifying and limiting exposure to asthma triggers, and treatment of other conditions that can worsen asthma, including allergic rhinitis, sinusitis, and reflux disease. The only medication in relation to which data are limited in pregnancy is leukotriene modifiers.

7

Taking control of asthma

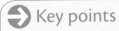 Key points

- Taking control is about empowering patients and parents to take important decisions regarding their or their children's asthma, with the aim of promoting good health, and preventing and treating exacerbation

- The key aspects are patient education, which is provided in a structured way, and a written self-management action plan

- People with asthma should be aware of the early signs of a flare-up and be prepared to act quickly

- Asthma action plans use changes in symptoms and/or peak flow to determine what action needs to be taken to prevent an exacerbation

Good control of asthma is important for many reasons. It improves quality of life, preserves lung function, and reduces the risk of exacerbations and hospital admission. However, poor control of asthma is not uncommon. Look at these statistics:

- suboptimal care and poor adherence to treatment contributes to 69,000 hospital admissions and 4 million GP consultations annually in the UK;

- almost 75% of hospital admissions for asthma are avoidable;

- almost 40% of patients with asthma do not react appropriately when their symptoms worsen;

- over 50% of individuals admitted to hospital for asthma had symptoms for more than a week before they took action;

- as many as 60% of asthmatics are poor at judging their breathlessness.

It is therefore important for people with asthma to understand and manage their disease to reduce hospital visits and admissions. Self-management for asthma involves the patient making therapeutic, behavioural, and environmental adjustments in accordance with advice from healthcare professionals.

 Fact!

Asthmatics with a self-management plan have a reduced number of hospital admissions, visits to the doctor's surgery, and days off work and school, and have better asthma control.

Empowering patients

Providing patients with information about their disease and ways of assessing control is the key first step. This whole notion of empowerment follows a movement towards patient-focused care, whereby patients are treated as partners rather than passive recipients of health care. With the changing outlook about diseases, patients are themselves changing and with the availability of various resources including the Internet, most patients look forward to a greater involvement in their care. Asthma can be considered a good example of patient-centred care, where patients can have a large say in the management of their asthma.

 Fact!

Asthma patients trained as part of the 'expert patient programme' used fewer drugs, had better lung function, and were more likely to take their medication compared with those who were not trained.

Empowering patients to take control of their own care brings many benefits to both the patient and the healthcare system. To feel empowered, the patient not only needs to be equipped with an education and management plan, but also needs to believe that they have the ability to help themselves. They will then feel comfortable with having more power to take control of their asthma rather than leaving all the decisions to the professional. Therefore, an empowered patient will have received ongoing support to develop the attributes and responsibilities that allow them to be an equal partner in their asthma management.

Self-management of asthma

Self-management is a cultural challenge for the healthcare professional, because it involves empowering patients to control their own asthma. It also put a huge onus on the patient, because the success of the self-management plan relies on the patient's willingness to take decisions about their asthma care. Some patients may not like the idea of taking on their own management decisions. Hence, education and motivation of both the patient and the healthcare professional are important. The objective of asthma self-management is to make the patient aware of how to manage their asthma under expert guidance. The key aspects are patient education, which is provided in a structured way, and a written self-management action plan. Peak flow is monitored regularly and asthmatic individuals are made aware of their symptoms. This helps to keep their asthma under good control and to act early when a deterioration of their condition begins. Medical supervision and continuity of care are also critical to the success of a self-management plan.

Some dos and don'ts of asthma

Do:

- try to identify the triggers for asthma and avoid or control them;

- recognize the early signs of an asthma flare-up by monitoring symptoms and peak flow measurements;

- maintain proper cleanliness of the house by washing bedding, pillow cases, quilts, and bedspreads regularly;

- keep moisture to a minimum;

- keep all medications within reach and use them as advised;

- keep reliever medications handy for an emergency;

- contact the doctor or the emergency department if the asthma worsens despite adequate control measures;

- keep your asthma under good control if you are pregnant, when it is all the more important—remember that if you have difficulty breathing, the fetus also has difficulty breathing;

- if you have exercise-induced asthma, avoid cold air;

- eat healthily—there are no special diets for asthma;

- get a 'flu jab' every year.

Don't:

- deny the fact that you have asthma;

- stop using your preventer inhaler, even when you are well;

- give up on the asthma-management programme agreed with your doctor;

- smoke, because cigarette smoke can trigger an asthma attack;

- use 'over-the-counter' asthma medicines;

- let heartburn symptoms go untreated, which can also worsen asthma;

- use your rescue medicine more than twice a week regularly without telling your doctor.

Do infections cause asthma?

Most patients recognize that their asthma gets worse when they have flu or another viral respiratory infection. Some children only get asthma symptoms when they have flu. Asthma is not caused by the infection, but a viral infection can trigger symptoms of asthma. Some individuals are born with a tendency to develop asthma and a viral infection acts like a catalyst to uncover hidden asthma. Infections that lead to worsening of asthma are usually, but not always, caused by viruses. In childhood asthma, the majority of asthma flare-ups are caused by viruses, and in a research study almost 80% of children with asthma flare-ups had evidence of viruses in their body. The virus is usually cleared within a few days, but its consequence, i.e. the asthma flare-up, needs to be tackled. Antibiotic are not usually helpful in these situations, because they are effective against bacterial—but not viral—infections. Thus, if the doctor does not prescribe an antibiotic, do not be surprised.

 Fact!

The airways are swollen in an asthmatic person and the inflammation caused by infections makes the narrowing of the airways worse, leading to a flare-up.

Symptoms of infection

Symptoms of chest infections that can lead to worsening of asthma include the following:

- worsening breathlessness, coughing, and wheezing;

- coughing up increased amounts of mucus;

- yellow or green phlegm;

- fever or chills;

- fatigue and weakness;

- sore throat and/or pain when swallowing food;

- blocked nose, runny nose, headaches, sinus drainage, and pain along the cheekbones.

However, people with asthma can also get bacterial infections in the lungs (bronchitis or even pneumonia), which may need to be treated with antibiotics. These antibiotics do not have any effect on the long-term, underlying airway swelling in asthma. This needs to be treated with a preventer (anti-inflammatory) medication. Because the inflammation also causes tightening of the muscles around the airways and narrowing of the airways, it should also be treated with a reliever medication.

Long-term infection of the nasal sinuses (chronic sinusitis) in childhood is a bacterial infection that can be a very stubborn chronic trigger for asthma. In these children, sinus X-rays or scans may be required to diagnose the condition. Antibiotic treatment for 3–4 weeks or longer may be needed to eradicate these infections completely. Asthma may also be triggered by an ear infection or bronchitis, which would also require antibiotic therapy.

What is an asthma flare-up?

During an asthma attack or flare-up, the airway swelling gets worse, making it even harder to breathe. The lungs can also produce a lot of sticky mucus, which can block the airways. The muscles around the airways also tighten up, making the airways very narrow. The overall effect is difficulty in breathing. Some people say that it is like breathing through a straw. There is also a tight or painful feeling to the chest, a whistling sound while breathing (wheeze), and sometimes a cough. Flare-ups also can cause sweating or make the person feel like their heart is beating faster than normal.

The warning signs of worsening asthma include:

- increasing breathlessness;

- increased wheezing, cough, and mucus production;

- night-time asthma symptoms;

- increased use of reliever medications;

- an increase in symptoms of exercise-induced asthma;

- decreased peak flow readings.

There is no universally accepted definition of a flare-up or exacerbation of asthma. In simple terms, it is a distinct worsening of asthma, as assessed by a deterioration in symptoms or lung function, or both. Asthma flare-ups can be mild, moderate, severe, or life-threatening. Although the characteristics of a flare-up may differ in different subjects, depending on their own symptoms and lung-function profile, a broad view is presented in Table 7.1.

Table 7.1 Characteristics of an asthma flare-up

Type of flare-up	Symptoms	Peak flow readings	Treatment
Mild	Breathless while talking or exercising Still able to speak in sentences Cough and wheeze	70–85% of predicted level	Need for reliever medication
Moderate	Breathless with minor effort Unable to complete sentences due to breathlessness Loud wheezing and night-time awakenings	Between 50 and 70% of predicted level	Need repeated reliever medications May also need extra medication
Severe	Breathless, even at rest Able to say only a few words due to breathlessness Cough is often prominent, but wheeze may not be Anxiety mounts quickly Rapid heart rate and sweating	Less than 50% of predicted level	Symptoms do not respond to reliever medications Treatment needs to be initiated immediately (possibly in an emergency room)

Some groups of patients are more likely to have a severe flare-up and even the risk of death. These patients should be particularly vigilant and be prepared to act quickly, before their asthma deteriorates to dangerous levels. These patients are characterized by:

- a history of sudden severe asthma worsening;

- previous use of a breathing machine for asthma flare-up;

- prior admission to an intensive care unit for asthma;

- two or more hospitalizations for asthma in the past year;

- three or more emergency-care visits for asthma in the past year;

- hospitalization or an emergency-care visit for asthma within the past month;

- use of more than two canisters per month of an inhaled, short-acting bronchodilator;

- current use of, or recent withdrawal from, steroid tablets;

- problems perceiving breathing difficulty or its severity;

- associated problems such as heart disease or smoking-induced lung disease;

- low socio-economic status and urban residence;

- illicit drug use;

- sensitivity to certain moulds such as *Alternaria*.

Managing asthma flare-ups

The most important aspect of managing an asthma attack is spotting the early clues to a flare-up. People with asthma are usually aware of worsening symptoms, but this can be an issue in those who are poor perceivers of symptoms. Here, it is useful to have a peak flow meter to check peak flows. If there is evidence of a flare-up, reliever medications should be used immediately. However, the patient should be aware of how much reliever medication is safe to use. This is something that will have been discussed by the doctor or asthma nurse. It is important for the patient to go through the personalized written action plan.

Table 7.2 A generic asthma action plan based on peak flow

Peak flow value	Level of asthma control	Action
Greater than 85% of personal best	Under control	Use regular treatment as advised
Less than 85% of personal best	Getting worse	Double the dose of inhaled steroids
Less than 70% of personal best	Exacerbation	Start course of oral prednisone (usually six tablets of 5 milligrams each)
Less than 50% of personal best	Emergency	Go to emergency room immediately

 Fact

Monitoring peak flows during a flare-up can provide pointers to improvement or worsening of symptoms. If symptoms are not improving or if peak flows are less than 50% of the expected level, call the doctor or go to the emergency room.

Self-management action plan

The doctor will prepare a self-management action plan detailing adjustments to the patient's medications based on their asthma symptoms and/or peak flow meter readings, or both. The development of individualized asthma action plan is the key to success in empowering patients to take control of their asthma. There are different action limits in the self-management plans (Table 7.2). Action plans provide patients and their families with information about when and how to use routine and emergency treatment, and how to monitor the disease. Asthma nurses provide support with self-management and continue to empower the patient, and their family and carers, to handle their condition as effectively as possible.

Why is a self-management action plan needed in asthma?

A self-management action plan is helpful in the treatment of asthma for the following reasons:

- asthma is a disease with wide variability in the symptoms, despite being on the correct medications;

- asthma worsening may lead to a hospital visit or admission, which could be prevented with correct treatment;

- more than half of people with asthma react inappropriately to asthma worsening;

- almost 30–40% of asthmatics do not use their inhaled medications as advised;

- some people with asthma are poor perceivers of their symptoms;

- self-management action plans have been shown to be effective in asthma management;

- self-management action plans have been shown to be cost-effective.

Setting up a self-management action plan

A plan can assist greatly in knowing what to do during an increase in symptoms (an acute worsening). If there is any doubt about what to do during an acute asthma exacerbation, the patient should contact their doctor. A patient who has a good understanding of asthma self-management should be able to:

- understand that asthma is a long-term treatable disease;

- describe their asthma symptoms and the treatment;

- participate in the control and management of their asthma;

- identify triggering factors;

- recognize signs of their asthma worsening;

- follow a written plan;

- use an inhaler correctly;

- take action to prevent and treat their asthma in different situations;

- address problems with compliance regarding the treatment;

- monitor symptoms and understand the objective measures of asthma control.

Content of a written asthma self-management plan

The basic details of the plan should include the date, patient's name, and their doctor's contact details. Some also include contact details for the patient's carer or emergency contact person. There may be some differences in different asthma action plans according to individuals' needs, but all plans should have some essential features. These include the following:

- it should be in a written format;

- it should be individualized for the patient, rather than a general example;

- it should contain information that allows the patient and/or their carer to recognize asthma worsening or a flare-up;

- it should contain information on what actions to take in response to these exacerbations.

Many plans follow a traffic light system for assessing the level of asthma control and provide early warnings of exacerbations. This moves from green (good control), through yellow (prepare to take action), to red (emergency) depending on the predefined frequency and severity of asthma symptoms and/or peak flow readings. Whichever system is used, the response plan needs to cover the following:

- maintenance/preventer therapy: doses and frequencies of regular medications;

- managing increased severity of symptoms: how to adjust treatment in response to particular signs and symptoms;

- treating exacerbations: when to start oral corticosteroids and seek medical advice;

- danger signs: when and how to seek urgent medical help.

The level of symptoms that indicate worsening may vary from individual to individual depending on their background control. Similarly, when peak expiratory flow (PEF) is used as a measure, this should be based on the patient's personal best (the best peak flow achieved by the patient), rather than a value predicted for age, height, and sex. PEF measurements in an asthma action plan can be beneficial for people with more severe or difficult-to-control asthma, and for those who do not perceive symptoms of deteriorating asthma control. Care should be taken when increasing treatment for a fall in PEF if there are no symptoms, because there is a risk of overtreatment. Reliance on PEF measurements is not recommended for children under 12 years. In most children with asthma, a change in symptoms is as effective as a PEF change for indicating that asthma is getting worse.

Interventions and self-management plans

Providing the self-management plan (Figure 7.1) to the patient puts the patient at the forefront of their asthma management. This type of self-management plan is particularly useful for patients who have moderate to severe asthma, have variable disease, been in the emergency department for asthma flare-ups, have poor perception of their asthma symptoms, and are keen and cooperative in taking up the advice.

Name: _____   Doctor/Nurse Conatct Number: _____
Best Peak Flow and Date taken: _____   Next of Kin: _____
Current Medications : _____

GREEN ZONE	YELLOW ZONE	YELLOW ZONE	RED ZONE
Peak flow above _____ (85% of best)	Peak flow between _____ and _____ (Between 70% and 85%)	Peak flow between _____ and _____ (Between 50% and 70%)	Peak flow less than _____
No or Minimal symptoms	Using reliever more than once daily	Using reliever every 4 hours or more frequently	Reliever not helping
Can do all normal activities	Difficulty with sleeping		Too breathless to sleep
Use preventer medication daily	Increase preventer medications	Continue preventer medication as in previous zone	Take reliever inhaler every minute for 5 minutes.
Name _____	Name _____	Take steroid tablets	If symptoms do not improve call 999 or a doctor immediately
Colour _____ Dose _____	Colour _____ Dose _____	Dose _____ mg (prednisolone) for _____ days or till symptoms better or peak flows at _____ for 2 days	
Number of Puffs _____	Number of Puffs _____	Inform the doctor or nurse	
Use reliever medications if having symptoms	Stay on the above dose until no symptoms for _____ days and then return to green zone	Use reliever medications as needed	
Name _____	Use reliever medications as needed	Name _____	
Colour _____ Dose _____	Name _____	Colour _____ Dose _____	
Number of Puffs _____	Colour _____ Dose _____	Number of Puffs _____	
	Number of Puffs _____		

Figure 7.1 An example of an asthma patient self-management plan.

8

Childhood asthma

➜ Key points

♦ Asthma often starts early in childhood; however, it is difficult to differentiate asthma from transient, viral infection-induced wheezing at this age

♦ The principles of management of childhood asthma are similar to those of adult asthma, but important differences exist in the choice of drugs and inhaler devices

♦ Asthma follows a course of remission and relapse during childhood, but can improve in the teenage years in nearly 50% of asthmatics

♦ Asthma is more common in boys during childhood, but changes at the time of puberty mean that it becomes more common and more severe in women

In the UK, over 1.1 million children (one in ten) are currently receiving treatment for asthma. In the USA, an estimated 6.5 million children under the age of 18 (nearly 1.4 million under the age of 5) have asthma. Underdiagnosis is not a huge problem now, but it is estimated that these figures may still underestimate the true prevalence. In the USA in 2003, asthma was the most common cause of school absenteeism due to a chronic disease. Asthma in children is more common among boys than girls. At least one child in seven will have 'wheezing' during their first five years. However, wheezing is even more common during the first two years of life. This is called early childhood wheeze and most of these children will not go on to have asthma in later childhood.

Fact!

A survey of 10-year-old children showed that almost 40% have wheezed at some point in their life.

Asthma in early childhood (aged <5 years)
Wheezing and asthma

Asthma is a chronic disease of the lungs that causes the airways to swell, tighten, and produce excess mucus. Wheezing is a high-pitched whistling sound that occurs when air is forced through the narrowed breathing tubes due to swelling of the lining of the airways, excessive secretions, or contraction of the airway muscles. Wheezing is common in children, however, it is important to know what parents mean when they report wheezing. In an interesting study, parents of 92 children with noisy breathing were asked to describe the sound: 53% described the noisy breathing as a 'wheeze'. They were then showed a video that described different lung sounds and asked whether they would like to revise their earlier description. Only 36% of the parents stuck to the original description of wheezing! However, it is difficult to assess lung function in small children and the diagnosis relies on parental reports of recurrent wheezing. It is therefore important to get an accurate description of the sound. It should also be remembered that wheezing can be caused by other conditions. For these reasons, it can be difficult to diagnose asthma with confidence, in children under the age of 5.

 Fact!

Wheezing can be caused by conditions other than asthma; hence, 'all who wheeze do not have asthma'.

The mechanics of babies' lungs also complicate the situation. Infants have a very small airway diameter, and even mild respiratory infections or exposure to irritants such as cigarette smoke can cause enough swelling of the inner lining (mucosa) to partially block the airways leading to obstruction and wheezing. Thus, coughing and wheezing develops in many infants—the typical symptoms of asthma. Among these are, of course, infants with true asthma. Studies have shown that infants who develop recurrent episodes of severe wheezing are most likely to go on to develop asthma, whilst those with mild or isolated episodes are more likely to grow out of it.

What causes recurrent wheezing?

Viral infections are the most common cause of recurrent wheezing in infants. The most commonly implicated virus is respiratory syncytial virus (RSV). Almost all children are exposed to this virus by the age of 2 years. In some children, infection by RSV can lead to narrowing of the airways causing wheezing. Viral infection can occur more than once, leading to recurrent wheezing. There are other factors that may increase the risk of wheezing in infants. They fall into three main groups as follows.

1. Infections and irritants:

    ◆ having siblings and/or attending day care (increased exposure to infection);

    ◆ maternal smoking (irritant exposure);

    ◆ low income and poor housing conditions (irritant exposure).

2. Developmental:

    ◆ low birth weight of the child (smaller bronchial tubes);

    ◆ male gender (smaller bronchial tubes);

    ◆ no breast feeding (child deprived of protective factors from the mother).

3. Allergy-related:

    ◆ parental allergy (genetic risk);

    ◆ other allergic disease such as eczema or food allergy (genetics and immune function);

    ◆ presence of pets and cockroaches (allergen exposure).

The increased risk of wheezing due to exposure to infections and irritants, including having siblings and daycare attendance, is confined to early childhood. Later, having siblings and attending daycare might actually be protective of asthma. Similarly, breastfeeding is protective against wheezing only in the first two years of life. There are several reasons for this. Breastfed infants get fewer viral infections due to protective antibodies in the breast milk. The immune system also develops better in breastfed babies due to nutritional factors present in the breast milk. However, this protective effect is lost as the child gets older.

Factors that increase infantile wheezing

- Maternal smoking during pregnancy

- Low birth weight

- Parental allergy

- Pets

- Lack of breast feeding

- Maternal asthma

- Caregiver skills and anxiety

- Crowded housing conditions

- Low income and socio-economic status

- Male gender

- Other siblings

- Daycare

Transient early wheezing

Almost 60% of infants and young children who wheeze grow out of it by the age of 6. This is why it is called transient early wheezing, i.e. an early life wheeze that does not persist. A typical example would be a bottle-fed boy, whose mother smokes. He may be living with his brother and sisters at home, and may attend a daycare centre. He would get repeated viral respiratory infections with recurrent wheezing, and his lung function, if measured, would be reduced. He is not allergic and would not show any effect of this wheezing in later childhood (once he had grown out of it), except perhaps for a mild reduction in lung function. Of course, not every child with early transient wheezing conforms to this example. However, infants with these characteristics have a higher risk of transient early wheezing that will improve with age.

Persistent wheezing

About 40% of all children who wheeze during the first three years of life continue to wheeze at 6 years of age. They are called persistent wheezers and the majority of these will be diagnosed as having asthma. Some of these are allergic children. They often have a family history of asthma and allergy, and may have other allergic disorders (eczema, food allergy, or rhinitis). About half of these persistent wheezers are sensitized to allergens by the age of 6 and the majority by the age of 10. Non-allergic persistent wheezers may be those children who had RSV infection during infancy. RSV infection increases the risk of asthma (and hence the wheezing persists), but not allergy.

 Fact!

Allergic asthma can start at any age, but most children develop their first symptoms before 6 years of age.

Can we predict which children will develop asthma?

Parents are often worried when their child wheezes, especially if it happens more than once or frequently. They want to know if their child is likely to continue to wheeze or improve and become a non-wheezer. If the persistence of wheezing can be predicted confidently, then it might be possible to take steps to prevent the development of asthma in infants who are at high risk. We know that among the larger group of infants who wheeze, 60–70% will improve and 30–40% will continue and become asthmatic. At present, it is not possible to predict with high accuracy, but children are at higher risk if they have:

◆ an asthmatic mother;

◆ recurrent chest infections in early childhood;

◆ a positive skin test to common allergens;

◆ atopic eczema and/or hay fever.

Children with all of the above characteristics will have an 80–90% risk of wheeze persistence and asthma development in later childhood, whilst those without any of the above characteristics will have a less than 10% risk.

The other question is whether, if a wheezy infant later develops asthma, we can predict whether it will be mild or severe. Again, we cannot be sure, but factors indicating severity of asthma in later childhood are:

◆ more frequent wheezing;

◆ early onset of wheezing (before 3 years of age);

◆ early onset of allergic sensitization (before 3 years of age).

Diagnosing asthma in infants

Diagnosing asthma in infants may be difficult. In older children and adults, breathing tests (lung function tests) can be used to make a confident diagnosis. However, these tests are less practical in very young children, because they require cooperation and understanding to get good results. Children usually do not develop these skills until they are about 5 years old. Some specialized breathing tests are possible, but they are mostly used in research. Instead, diagnosis is usually made following clinical assessment. The signs and symptoms of asthma in young children include:

◆ breathing problems—loud wheezy breathing and/or faster breathing;

◆ intermittent wheezing with prolonged symptom-free periods;

◆ frequent coughing or cough worsening after play;

◆ wheezing brought on by vigorous laughing or crying;

◆ difficulty eating or suckling;

◆ lethargy;

◆ quieter-than-normal crying.

Treatment of wheezy babies

All wheezy infants behave in the same way, and it is not possible to differentiate confidently between those who will later develop asthma and those who will improve. Therefore, the approach to treatment is the same for both groups. The wheezing episodes are treated by reliever medication administered by an inhaler attached to a spacer and a mask. Nebulizers are also used, but an inhaler attached to a spacer works equally effectively. Attacks that are not relieved by inhalers may need a short course of steroid tablets. If the child continues to have recurrent attacks, then a trial of preventer medications should be considered. Inhaled steroids are effective as the first-line treatment. Other medications such as the leukotriene modifier montelukast (see Chapter 6) may be tried, if the wheezing is not well controlled. Side effects are uncommon, but one concern regarding inhaled steroids is reduction in height as an adult. However, studies have shown that children who have used inhaled steroids for a long period will attain the same height as their peers, although there maybe a delayed growth spurt.

 Case study

Wheezy child

A 2-year-old baby was brought in by her parents because she was having breathing difficulties. The baby was found to have had a wheeze for the past week. She had a similar episode six months previously, which was mild and settled without treatment. She had been unwell for a few weeks and had developed the wheeze recently. There was no history of asthma, allergies, hay fever, or eczema in the family. The baby's chest X-ray was normal. A swab from the nose of the child showed the presence of respiratory syncytial virus (RSV). The baby was provided with a reliever inhaler and her symptoms improved. She was also given low-dose inhaled steroids. The symptoms were effectively controlled, but the parents were worried that she would develop asthma later in life. She is now 8 years old, completely off her medications, and is fit and well with no symptoms suggestive of asthma.

Asthma in older children (aged 5–12 years)

Asthma in children is similar to asthma in adults in the sense that they have similar triggering factors, a similar profile of inflammation in the airways, and similar symptoms. However, there are various features that are specific to childhood asthma. It affects more boys than girls and is usually due to allergy. There are also important considerations to make in the management. Optimal treatment of airway inflammation not only improves symptoms, but may also prevent irreversible damage to the airways later in life. However, this needs to be balanced against possible concerns over side effects, especially of inhaled steroids, and particularly on growth and susceptibility to infection.

Fact!

Although asthma cannot be cured, it can almost always be controlled.

Thus, it is important to have a correct diagnosis and to be on the correct medications to control asthma. In children aged 5 and over, it is possible to get a good history and to carry out lung function tests. Therefore, the criteria for diagnosis are similar to those used in adults:

◆ typical symptoms (cough, wheeze, chest tightness, and shortness of breath);

◆ obstruction of airway passages in lung function tests;

◆ improvement in airway obstruction on its own or with treatment;

◆ day-to-day changes in symptoms and lung function.

Inhaled mediations are the cornerstone of asthma treatment. Inhaled steroids are generally safe, because most children respond to treatment at low doses. Only a minority require high doses of inhaled steroids. Maintenance treatment with inhaled steroids controls asthma symptoms, improves the quality of life, lung function, and airway sensitivity, and reduces the frequency of acute exacerbations and the number of hospital admissions. However, inhaled steroids do not cure asthma. Inflammation (and symptoms) returns quickly (within days to weeks) if inhaled steroid treatment is stopped.

Almost all children can be taught how to use inhalers effectively, but the choice of inhaler should depend on the child (Table 8.1). The choice of inhaler device should include consideration of the efficacy of drug delivery, cost, safety,

Table 8.1 Inhaler devices for children with asthma

Age group	Preferred device	Alternative device
Younger than 4 years	Metered-dose inhaler with spacer and a face mask	Nebulizer with face mask
Aged 4–6 years	Metered-dose inhaler with spacer and mouthpiece	Nebulizer with mouthpiece
Older than 6 years	Dry-powder inhaler, breath-activated inhaler, or metered-dose inhaler with spacer and mouthpiece	Nebulizer with mouthpiece

ease of use, convenience, and documentation of its use in the patient's age group. In general, the choices are:

- a metered-dose inhaler used through a spacer;

- a dry-powder inhaler;

- a breath-activated inhaler;

- a nebulizer.

Spacers retain large drug particles that would normally be deposited in the mouth and throat, reducing the side effects of the inhaled drug. Nebulizers have a rather imprecise dosing, and are expensive, time-consuming to use and care for, and require maintenance. They are mainly reserved for children who cannot use other inhaler devices. During an asthma attack, a nebulizer is often used, although a metered-dose inhaler with a spacer is equally effective.

Stepwise management

The principles of the management of childhood asthma are similar to those used for adults albeit with minor modifications (Figure 8.1). Following diagnosis, the step at which treatment is initiated depends on the severity of asthma. Once control has been achieved and maintained for at least three months, treatment can be stepped down. If control is not satisfactory, treatment can be stepped up. If a child with previously diagnosed asthma is seen, the treatment recommended will depend on the current level of asthma control. If the asthma is not controlled on the current treatment regimen, treatment should be stepped up until control is achieved. If control has been maintained for at least three months, treatment can be stepped down with the aim of establishing the lowest step and dose of treatment that maintains control. The five steps of treatment are as follows.

1. Step 1 is treatment only with a reliever inhaler and is reserved for those with occasional symptoms of short duration:

   - daytime: twice or less a week;

   - night-time: once a week or less.

2. Step 2 involves regular preventer medication. This is usually low-dose inhaled steroids. Alternatives to inhaled steroids are:

   - leukotriene modifiers (such as montelukast) as a tablet;

   - sodium cromoglicate inhaler.

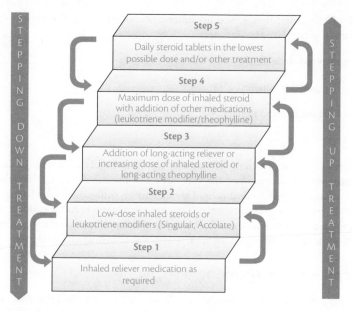

Figure 8.1 Stepwise management of asthma in children.

3. Step 3 of treatment recommends either:

- a combination of a low-dose of inhaled steroid with an inhaled long-acting bronchodilator (separately as two inhalers or combined into one inhaler);

or

- an increase to a medium dose of inhaled steroids.

4. Step 4 has the following options available in sequence:

- combine a medium dose of inhaled steroid with a long-acting inhaled bronchodilator;

- add a leukotriene modifier (such as montelukast);

- add theophylline;

- increase the dose of inhaled steroid further.

5. Step 5 of management involves the addition of steroid tablets at the lowest dose required to control asthma.

The course of asthma in children

In an individual asthmatic, asthma may follow a relapsing and remitting course throughout childhood. The ongoing presence of airway inflammation is the key factor for relapse and remissions in asthma. Thus, the course largely depends on the underlying severity of asthma and how well it is treated.

Mild asthma

This may improve for long periods when preventer treatment may not be required and symptoms may occur only occasionally, for example following strenuous exercise or a viral infection. However, any reduction in asthma medication, e.g. discontinuation of the preventer inhaler, should not be done without the prior agreement and knowledge of the treating doctor or asthma nurse.

Moderate asthma

If well treated, asthma does not cause problems in day-to-day life. Remission is less common, but can occur. If the asthma remains well controlled with few symptoms, a step down in treatment is justified and should be attempted following discussion with the doctor. However, a major problem in this group of patients is inadequate and intermittent treatment of underlying inflammation, whereby asthmatic children stop using their preventer inhaler because their symptoms have improved, only to find that their asthma relapses later with a vengeance.

Severe asthma

The primary goal of treatment of asthma is to control symptoms and to lead a normal life. This is easier said than done in these individuals, who may not be symptom-free, despite being on the right treatment and using their medications as advised. This is a small group (less than 5% of all asthmatics), but one that requires special attention. In this group, the aim is to control symptoms as much as possible and to reduce the number of asthma attacks, thereby preventing emergency visits and hospital admissions.

Asthma in adolescence (aged 12–17 years)

A major problem during the years of adolescence is compliance with medication. This is partly to do with natural behaviour of the adolescents and partly due to the actual improvement observed in asthma symptoms in many patients at this stage in life. This is known as 'growing out of asthma'. As a result, many teenagers stop using their inhalers. Teenagers, with their natural feelings of invincibility, compounded with the fact that many of their peers have successfully given up inhalers, unwisely stop taking their treatment. These adolescents are at highest risk of asthma attacks and even death. A reduction in medication should only be done as a planned stepping down of treatment, under medical supervision, in patients in whom asthma actually improves. Studies have highlighted some features that indicate whether asthma is likely to continue to cause problems through adolescence (see box below). Those who do not have these characteristic have a very good chance of their asthma going into remission, but an increased number of these features indicates an increased risk of asthma persisting.

Risk factors for asthma persistence in adolescence

- Early onset of asthma

- Severity of asthma

- Reduced lung function

- A family history of asthma

- Having another allergic disease such as atopic eczema or rhinitis

- Allergic sensitization

- Smoking

- Being female

- Obesity

Most of these risk factors are easily explained. It is understandable that those with early onset of persistent and severe asthma are more likely to continue to have symptoms. Similarly, adolescents who have a family history of asthma or are allergic (having atopic eczema, rhinitis, or allergic sensitization) are likely to be at high risk of persistence due to the genes they carry or continued allergen exposure. Smoking is another obvious risk factor that is likely to prevent remission. Therefore, adolescents with asthma must never start smoking, even for a short period or intermittently, under peer pressure. The last two factors are worth mentioning in more detail. These are being female and obesity.

Female gender

Asthma is more common in boys throughout childhood. A gender reversal is observed during adolescence, with asthma prevalence in females surpassing that in males. Because this gender reversal occurs at the same time that asthma seems to improve in many children, there are several interesting possibilities to explain this:

- asthma improves in boys, but persist in girls;

- asthma improves equally in both sexes, but new asthma develops in girls during adolescence;

- a combination of the above two explanations.

We do not know exactly what happens, but studies are being done to investigate this further.

Another interesting fact is that severe asthma is much more common in women then men. Overall, asthma is twice as common in women as it is in men. However, severe asthma is several times more common in women. Interestingly, this severe asthma is often non-allergic. We do not know why women get more asthma than men and why it is more severe. However, it is obvious that this change occurs during adolescence. One study showed that reduced growth in lung function due to asthma occurred in females, but not males, during the teen years. This may be to do with pubertal hormonal changes. At least one study has shown that early puberty in women may increase the risk of asthma persistence in women. Deposition of fat is one of the natural changes that occur at the time of puberty in women, but not in men, leading to the question of whether this fat deposition contributes to the increase in asthma in women.

 Fact!

Asthma in younger children is more common in boys, but a gender reversal occurs at puberty, so that asthma becomes more common in older girls and women.

Asthma and obesity

In recent years, there has been considerable interest in the relationship between obesity and asthma. It has been argued by some that obese subjects complain of shortness of breath because they are not fit and that this may mistakenly be diagnosed as asthma. However, obese subjects with a diagnosis of asthma have been shown to have airways obstruction in tests on pulmonary function. Some also argue that obesity does not cause asthma; rather, it is actually asthma that causes obesity in children who are unwilling or unable to participate in physical activities, because they get exercise-induced asthma. However, this was not the case when children were analysed in a longitudinal birth cohort study. If this argument was correct, then children diagnosed with asthma at the age of 4 should have become obese by the age of 10. This was not the case. Indeed, no link was found between asthma and obesity in children from birth up to 10 years of age. Many other studies have supported this view that the link between asthma and obesity develops at puberty in teenage girls, and is then seen primarily in women. Additionally, obesity may also increase the severity of asthma, so that weight reduction improves asthma symptoms and lung function. Can obesity, therefore, explain the higher prevalence and more severe asthma seen in women? This is an interesting possibility. At present, we do not know if female obesity, acquired during adolescence, explains all or some of the gender effect, but further research is being carried out.

 Fact!

The link between obesity and asthma develops in teenage girls, and is then observed primarily in women.

Natural history of asthma

We know that in many children asthma may improve for long periods and sometimes a cure is presumed. However, in some of these children (in whom a cure has been presumed), asthma does return. Also, asthma may start at any time during childhood (or, less commonly, in adult life). Asthma evolves through the following stages from infancy to early adult life.

Early childhood (aged <5 years)

As described above, the majority of early life wheezers improve and for this reason they are often not labelled as having asthma.

Later childhood

Some early life wheezers continue (persistent wheezers) and are diagnosed as asthmatic. To this pool are added children who start to wheeze in later childhood (between 5 and 10 years of age). These are called late onset asthmatics. Thus, early onset persistent wheezers and late onset asthmatics form the bulk of children who suffer from asthma during childhood.

Adolescence

During this period (aged 12–17 years), 50% of asthmatic children improve to the extent that they are able to give up their preventer inhalers and do not often need their reliever inhalers. It is in these situations that asthma is often presumed to be cured and, in many cases, it does go away for good.

Relapse after remission

Unfortunately, a relapse can occur after a remission during adolescence. Thus, 30–50% of asthmatic subjects who have apparently grown out of asthma during adolescence develop symptoms again in early adult life (aged 18–30 years). It is therefore important to follow up asthma patients who are in remission to detect any signs of relapse and initiate early treatment. At present, we cannot confidently predict who will have a relapse. However, people with reduced lung function in childhood have an increased risk of relapse if they go into remission. People with childhood asthma should certainly avoid smoking and should perhaps avoid going into professions with higher levels of occupational exposure to certain allergens. However, a history of asthma in remission should not be used as an excuse to prejudice employment opportunities for young adults.

 Fact!

Almost 50% of adolescents who grow out of asthma relapse in early adulthood.

Summary

In summary, childhood asthma is common and there are important differences with regard to its natural history and management compared with adult asthma. It should be remembered that asthma often starts in childhood, and asthma seen in adult life is often a continuation or relapse of childhood asthma, although occasionally asthma can start in adult life. The principles of management are similar, with emphasis on avoidance of allergens and irritants, and regular anti-inflammatory treatment. Monitoring of compliance and side effects is of the utmost importance. Although a cure is not possible, remission often occurs as the child grows, especially if the asthma was well controlled in childhood and lung function has been preserved.

9

Asthma and other allergic diseases

> **→ Key points**
>
> ◆ Hay fever, eczema, and food allergy often coexist with asthma in the same individual
>
> ◆ In those with asthma and hay fever, optimal treatment of hay fever will help to improve asthma control
>
> ◆ A food allergy may trigger asthma, but this happens in a relatively small subgroup of asthmatics
>
> ◆ Children with eczema in early childhood have a higher risk of developing asthma and hay fever in later childhood and adolescence

Asthma, hay fever, food allergy, and atopic eczema are related allergic conditions, and have a tendency to cluster in individuals and families. This is due to the fact that these diseases are caused by allergic mechanisms that originate in the genes that these individual or families share. Typically, a child born with this allergic tendency may develop food allergy and eczema in early childhood, which is replaced by respiratory allergies (asthma and/or hay fever) in later childhood. This progression of allergic diseases during childhood has been given the term 'allergic march'.

Asthma and hay fever

Strictly speaking, hay fever is defined as an allergic reaction to grass or hay pollen. However, when this condition is due to allergy to tree, weed, or flower pollen, it is also called hay fever, and this term is often used even when symptoms occur all year round as a result of allergy to dust mites, animals, or moulds. The correct term for pollen allergic disease is seasonal allergic rhinitis, because the pollen exposure is seasonal, depending on the type of pollen and geographical area. The grass pollen season is between May and July. Tree pollens are released earlier (March–May) and certain weeds are released later in the year (July–September). The offending allergen is different in different countries and depends on the prevailing pollen in a particular geographic region. The major causes of hay fever throughout the world are:

- grass pollen in the UK;

- ragweed in the USA;

- birch tree pollen in Scandinavia;

- cedar pollen in Japan.

A pollen calendar provides information on the pollens in a particular area (Figure 9.1). Asthma and hay fever commonly occur together, and in these individuals, asthma symptoms can get worse during the pollen season. Adolescents and young adults with severe hay fever often get asthma symptoms during the pollen season, even if they have not been formally diagnosed with the condition.

 Fact!

Hay fever and asthma often coexist. If a child has hay fever, there is a higher chance that they will develop asthma later.

Hay fever affects 15% of the population in the UK. Regarded as trivial by the ignorant, hay fever varies from mild forms, which are indeed trivial, to a severity that can be crippling during the pollen season. Sufferers may be unable to work or drive, and it affects school and exam performance. Hay fever is very common and often first develops in the teenage years. Symptoms occur seasonally each year, but in many patients they improve with time, so that severe hay fever is less common in adults and the elderly. All-year-round hay fever, due to allergy to moulds, dust mites, and animal dander, is called perennial allergic rhinitis.

Symptoms of hay fever

The symptoms of hay fever are due to the body's immune system reacting to pollen. Cells on the lining of the nose and eyes release histamines and other substances that cause swelling of the linings of the nasal passages and the eyes

Generalised UK pollen & fungal spores calendar

The calenders below show the general pattern of allergenic pollen and fungal spore release in the UK. The exact timing and severity of pollen and spore seasons will vary from year to year depending on the weather, and also regionally depending on geographical location.

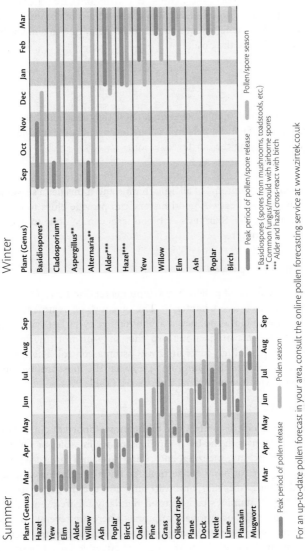

For an up-to-date pollen forecast in your area, consult the online pollen forecasting service at www.zirtek.co.uk between the months of April and September

Figure 9.1 Example of a pollen calendar for the UK. Reproduced with permission of the National Pollen and Aerobiology Research Unit, University of Worcester.

when they come in contact with pollen. This causes inflammation in the nose (rhinitis) and eyes (conjunctivitis). Symptoms in the nose include sneezing, runny nose, blocked nose, and itching. Eye symptoms are watering, itching, a gritty feeling, and redness and swelling of the whites of the eyes. Uncommon symptoms are headache, sweating, and facial pain, due to sinus involvement caused by swelling in the nose.

 Fact!

Asthma symptoms such as wheezing, chest tightness, and breathlessness can get worse when the person has hay fever and some individuals have asthma only during the hay fever season.

If the person has symptoms of allergic rhinitis and if this has a seasonal profile, then the diagnosis is easy. A good history can provide clues to the diagnosis and the likely triggers. Skin tests or blood tests can be done to determine the specific allergic triggers.

Treatment of hay fever

It is impossible to avoid pollen, but symptoms tend to be less severe if pollen exposure is reduced (see Chapter 5). The objective of treatment is to be able to lead a normal life. It is not necessary to remove every last symptom, only to make the symptoms mild enough so that they do not interfere with life. Effective treatment of hay fever improves asthma control. The treatment will depend on how severe the symptoms are, what the most troublesome symptoms are, and what the individual's needs are (Table 9.1).

Antihistamines

Antihistamines block histamine, one of the most important chemicals mediating allergic responses in the body. Antihistamines in tablet or syrup form are useful for nasal itching, sneezing, and runny nose, and for eye symptoms, but are not as effective for nasal congestion. An antihistamine nasal spray rapidly eases nasal itching, sneezing, and watering, and eye drops are useful for eye symptoms. Antihistamines can be used regularly for frequent symptoms or 'as required' for mild, occasional symptoms. There are several brands of antihistamine that can be bought at pharmacies, but some are available only on prescription. Most of the new types are effective for 24 hours, which is convenient. A dose usually works within an hour.

Table 9.1 Commonly used treatment options for hay fever

Most troubling symptom	Most appropriate first treatment	Additional treatment
Nasal blockage and watering	Steroid nasal spray	Antihistamine tablets
Watery, itchy nose and sneezing; watery, itchy eyes	Antihistamine tablets	Cromoglicate or antihistamine eye drops
Watery, itchy nose, and sneezing	Antihistamine nasal spray	Steroid nasal spray
Nasal blockage in children	Cromoglicate nasal spray	Steroid nasal spray

 Fact!

Nearly all of the older antihistamines cause drowsiness. Newer ones cause less drowsiness. Antihistamines that cause drowsiness should not be used if driving or handling machinery.

Nasal steroid sprays

For those with symptoms on most days (or every day), the first-line treatment is nasal steroid sprays. Nasal corticosteroid sprays reduce and control the impact of many of the mediators that can cause inflammation in the nose. These medications improve all symptoms of allergic rhinitis, but are more effective on nasal blockage and runny nose. However, it may take several weeks in some patients for the nasal steroids to take full effect. They may not have any immediate effect on symptoms. It is best to start them 1–2 weeks prior to the start of the hay fever season. A steroid spray can be used in conjunction with antihistamines if the symptoms are not controlled by just one of the medications. Because the dose of steroids in the spray is small, they are unlikely to cause side effects. Occasionally, patients report nasal bleeding, in which case use of the nasal spray should be stopped.

 Fact!

Nasal steroids should be used regularly (every day) for optimal effect.

Other sprays

Like steroid sprays, sodium cromoglicate nasal sprays and eye drops take a while to build up their effect and they need to be taken regularly. Sodium cromoglicate is thought to work by stopping the release of histamine from cells (called mast cells). A disadvantage of this medication is that it needs to be taken 4–5 times a day.

Decongestants

Decongestant pills or sprays are occasionally used when nasal congestion cannot be relieved with other medications. They have an immediate effect of clearing a blocked nose. However, relief is often transient and symptoms tend to come back with a vengeance, requiring more frequent and higher doses of the medication with considerable potential for side effects. Decongestant tablets also improve the symptoms of nasal blockage, but have a number of side effects. Although these medications are available without prescription, they need to be used with caution.

 Fact!

Decongestant tablets are available without prescription, alone or in combination with antihistamines, and are effective, but they may have a number of side effects.

Oral steroids

Rarely, a short course of steroid tablets is prescribed for those with severe hay fever not responding to the standard treatment described above and if their school, exam, or work performance is being affected, for example, students sitting exams and having severe symptoms. Steroids usually work well to reduce inflammation. A short course is usually safe. However, this should not be taken for long periods to treat hay fever, because serious side effects may develop.

Allergen immunotherapy

Also known as allergy shots, allergen immunotherapy may be considered if symptoms persist despite standard treatment. Here, the allergen is given in increasing doses, starting with a very small dose, to induce tolerance to that allergen. The idea is to desensitize the individual to the offending allergen. The process takes 2–3 years to achieve full desensitization and is not useful if people are allergic to multiple allergens. In hay fever patients, the allergen used is a pollen or pollen mix. Traditionally, it involved a series of injections, but now the allergen can be given by drops or in tablet form, which dissolves under the tongue. This is the only treatment that continues to be effective after treatment is stopped. Immunotherapy treatment of hay fever also reduces the risk of later asthma development.

Treatment of asthma during the hay fever season

Asthma treatment may need to be increased in the hay fever season to counteract the effect of pollens. This can be done by increasing the dose of inhaled steroids or by adding a tablet medication that blocks the effect of leukotrienes (another chemical that mediates allergic inflammation). This medication, called montelukast (or zafirlukast), has the advantage of being effective for both asthma and hay fever.

 Fact!

If asthma becomes worse in the hay fever season, an increase in treatment may be needed. For those hay fever sufferers who get asthma symptoms only during the pollen season, a bronchodilator with or without a steroid inhaler may be needed.

Asthma and food allergy

Food allergy is one of many reasons why someone can react badly to a food. Food allergy is when immune system mistakenly recognizes the food or food components as harmful substances and reacts. There are also some adverse reactions to foods that involve the body's metabolism, but not the immune system. These reactions are known as food intolerance. Examples of food intolerance include the inability to digest certain food components properly, such as lactose (milk sugar). Allergic reactions to food occur in 1–7% of the population according to various estimates. They are more common in children, in whom over 90% of food allergy is caused by only eight foods. These are:

- dairy produce: milk and eggs;
- fish and shellfish;
- peanuts and tree nuts;
- wheat and sesame.

In some cases, the allergy may disappear as the child gets older. This is particularly likely to happen in infants and toddlers who suffer from cow's milk allergy, the commonest kind of food allergy to affect them. It is less likely when they acquire a nut or fish allergy. Signs and symptoms of food allergic reactions may include one or more of the following:

- itching/tingling/swelling of the lips, palate, tongue, or throat;

- skin reactions such as hives, skin rashes, itching, or flushing;

- nasal congestion or itchiness, a runny nose, or sneezing;

- itchy and streamy eyes;

- abdominal symptoms such as nausea, vomiting, colic, cramp-like pain, and diarrhoea;

- chest tightness, shortness of breath, or wheezing.

Does food allergy cause asthma?

Food allergy can cause asthma, but this is rare. Of course, any food allergic reaction may involve breathing difficulties and wheezing, i.e. an asthma-like condition, but this is transient and occurs only as part of the allergic/anaphylactic reaction. What is more controversial is if asthma is exacerbated or triggered by foods on a daily basis. Many asthmatics believe this to be the case. With the current state of knowledge, it can be said that foods may cause or trigger asthma in some children and probably even fewer adults. In the vast majority of allergic individuals, asthma is caused by inhaled allergens, such as dust mites. However, a small proportion of children with very severe asthma tend to have severe food allergies as well, such as peanut or nut allergy. It is possible that food allergies may make asthma worse in these children. It is also possible that children with severe asthma react badly to foods. There are four types of food that have been implicated in asthma, as follows.

1. Known and potent food allergens (such as milk, eggs, peanuts, tree nuts, soy, wheat, fish, and shellfish) have been found to trigger asthma, especially in those who are highly allergic. There is some concern that, in these children, minute amounts of food that get airborne may cause airway narrowing, e.g. if the food is being cooked in the kitchen or served on the table in the presence of the child.

2. Those with aspirin (salicylic acid)-sensitive asthma may react to salicylate occurring naturally in the foods. Certain foods, especially some fruits and

vegetables, are high in salicylate and these may trigger asthma in sensitive subjects.

3. Rarely, sulfites and sulfiting agents in foods (found in dried fruits, prepared potatoes, wine, bottled lemon or lime juice, and shrimps) trigger asthma.

4. Many food ingredients such as food dyes and colourings, and food preservatives including as butylated hydroxyanisole (BHA) and butylated hydroxytoluene (BHT), monosodium glutamate, aspartame, and nitrite, have been linked to asthma, but evidence to support this is not forthcoming.

However, it is important to be sure that food is causing or contributing to asthma. It is not uncommon to see a child's diet being unnecessarily restricted with a presumed diagnosis of food-induced asthma and as a result depriving the child of nutritional foods. The diagnosis of food-induced asthma should only be made following an appropriate allergy assessment.

 ## Case study

Asthma and allergy

An 11-year-old child was referred to an allergy clinic for assessment of his allergies. He had developed eczema and egg allergy at the age of 6 months. However, both his eczema and his egg allergy improved over the next two years. He then had an allergic reaction to peanut butter at the age of 3 years, which was the first time he was knowingly given peanuts. He has since strictly avoided peanuts and other nuts. At the age of 8 years, he developed wheezing and shortness of breath when participating in games at school. He was prescribed a reliever inhaler, which helped him. At the age of 10, he developed nasal blockage, sneezing, and a runny nose, and was referred to the allergy clinic. On questioning, he described regular symptoms of cough and wheeze, which had not previously been appreciated. Following an allergy test, he was found to be allergic to house dust mites and his nut allergy was also confirmed. His lung function was less than normal. He was given advice on allergen avoidance, and prescribed regular treatment for asthma and nasal allergy. When seen again three months later, he was much better, with normal lung function and only occasional symptoms.

Prevention of food-induced asthma

The best way to avoid food-induced asthma is to eliminate the offending food or food ingredient from the diet and, if necessary, from the environment. Reading ingredient information on food labels and knowing where food triggers of asthma are found are the best defences against a food-induced asthma attack. The main objectives of an asthmatic's care and treatment are to stay healthy, to remain symptom-free, to enjoy food, to be able to exercise, to use medications properly, and to follow the care plan developed between the doctor and the patient.

Asthma and eczema

Atopic eczema is a chronic, itchy skin condition in which the skin is dry and overly sensitive to many things, including common allergens. In young children, cows' milk and egg allergy may be causative, and exclusion can sometimes help to improve eczema. In older children and adults, house dust mites may be the cause. However, allergy is only one aspect of a complex set of risk factors and triggers that include infection and stress. There is no definitive way of predicting whether a child will develop eczema, but a parental history of eczema and atopy increases a child's risk, indicating a genetic component to the risk. This combined with environmental factors can cause eczema and, in some cases, allergic rhinitis or asthma.

A link exists between eczema and asthma. One study found that 46% of children with asthma also had eczema. Those with eczema in early childhood have a higher risk of developing asthma and hay fever later, and the common denominator seems to be a tendency to become sensitized to common food and inhalant allergens. Thus, avoidance of the allergen helps improve the symptoms of allergic diseases including asthma and eczema. There is also some evidence that strict avoidance of food and dust mite allergens in early infancy might prevent the development of asthma and eczema in those with high genetic risk.

Appendix

Asthma information websites

Asthma UK

Asthma UK is a charity dedicated to improving the health and well-being of the 5.2 million people in the UK whose lives are affected by asthma. Available at: http://www.asthma.org.uk.

British Lung Foundation

The British Lung Foundation is a UK charity working for everyone affected by lung disease. It focuses on resources providing support for people affected by lung disease and works in a variety of ways, including funding world-class research, to bring about positive change and to improve treatment, care, and support for people affected by lung disease, now and in the future. Available at: http://www.lunguk.org/.

British Thoracic Society

The British Thoracic Society is a registered charity, the objective of which is to improve the standards of care of people who have respiratory diseases. Its web pages also contain information of interest to people who have respiratory diseases and asthma, and there is useful information, as well as links to dedicated sites run by lung charities. Available at: http://www.brit-thoracic.org.uk.

Global Initiative for Asthma

The Global Initiative for Asthma (GINA) works with healthcare professionals and public-health officials around the world to reduce asthma prevalence, morbidity, and mortality. Resources such as evidence-based guidelines for asthma management provide plans for the management of asthma and, together with patient involvement and organizing events such as the annual celebration of World Asthma Day, GINA is working to improve the lives of people with asthma in every corner of the globe. Available at: http://www.ginasthma.com/.

The Anaphylaxis Campaign

The Anaphylaxis Campaign is an independent charity guided by leading UK allergists. It provides patient information on various allergies and methods of avoiding allergies. Available at: http://www.anaphylaxis.org.uk.

Allergy UK

Allergy UK is a registered charity that provides up-to-date information on all aspects of allergy, food intolerance, and chemical sensitivity. There is a wealth of allergy information available on this site, including many detailed fact sheets and articles written and approved by leading specialists in the field of allergy. Available at: http://www.allergyuk.org/.

European Federation of Asthma and Allergy Associations

The European Federation of Asthma and Allergy Associations (EFA) is an alliance of 27 organizations in 14 different countries across Europe. The EFA is a European network of patient organizations that was founded in 1991, prompted by the belief that an international organization formed by European patient associations that share the same aims would be a more effective way of serving the needs and safeguarding the rights of patients and their carers. Available at: http://www.efanet.org.

Index